Epidemiology with R

Epidemiology with R

BENDIX CARSTENSEN

Steno Diabetes Center Copenhagen, Gentofte and
Department of Biostatistics,
University of Copenhagen, Denmark

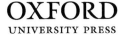
OXFORD
UNIVERSITY PRESS

OXFORD
UNIVERSITY PRESS

Great Clarendon Street, Oxford, OX2 6DP,
United Kingdom

Oxford University Press is a department of the University of Oxford.
It furthers the University's objective of excellence in research, scholarship,
and education by publishing worldwide. Oxford is a registered trade mark of
Oxford University Press in the UK and in certain other countries

First Edition published in 2021
Impression: 2

Published in the United States of America by Oxford University Press
198 Madison Avenue, New York, NY 10016, United States of America

British Library Cataloguing in Publication Data
Data available

Library of Congress Control Number: 2020942510

ISBN 978–0–19–884132–6 (hbk.)
ISBN 978–0–19–884133–3 (pbk.)

DOI: 10.1093/oso/9780198841326.001.0001

Printed and bound by
CPI Group (UK) Ltd, Croydon, CR0 4YY

Contents

Preface

At the R-project website it says that 'R is a free software environment for statistical computing and graphics.'

The foundation for any type of statistical computing (and indeed any endeavour in so-called 'data science') is a *statistical model*. Which may not always be explicit; almost any computing on data implicitly assumes some sort of probability model or, more precisely, a set of models—occasionally different models may lead to the same computations.

If we, for example, compute a mortality rate by taking the number of deaths and divide by the amount of person-years, we are implicitly working with a model assuming that the mortality rate is constant over the observation period. This is because the constant mortality model yields the ratio of deaths to person-years as the estimator of the constant mortality rate. People may argue that they assumed nothing; they just divided the numbers to get an 'overall figure'. But the resulting number only makes sense in the constant mortality model.

In this book I have tried to be explicit about model assumptions. So (almost) all computations will be based on some explicitly defined model.

In order to move from a probability model that we assume generated data, to statistical inference (going from data to model instead), a principle for estimation of the parameters governing the probability machinery is required. The most commonly used is the maximum likelihood principle, which will be the only one used in this book. It has the advantage that it yields the classical intuitive estimators in virtually all simple situations.

Classical epidemiological texts mostly focus on comparing 'exposed' to 'non-exposed' individuals with respect to some outcome such as lung cancer diagnosis or death. Which indeed is relevant, but it has had the (unintended?) effect of rendering the vast majority of epidemiological studies as group-comparison studies, where quantitative ('continuous') variables are grouped and a separate effect / parameter is estimated for each group. In this text I have tried to emphasize that laboriously collected data should be used to the greatest possible extent, and that grouping quantitative variables constitutes discarding information, and therefore should be avoided. Hence, the book emphasizes tools and examples that show how to exploit quantitative explanatory variables maximally, and in particular provide examples of graphical reporting of the effects of quantitative variables.

What this book is not

It is not a textbook on epidemiology, statistics, or data science. Basic principles underlying the models used are included in order to establish the rationale for the data structures and analysis tools. So it is a book that tries not only to explain 'how to' with R, but also 'why' a given function is used.

But you will, for example, find that the introduction of confounding is rudimentary, and that there is no mention of the machinery of causal inference. The book is intended to give the statistical background needed to understand the mechanics of the R code needed in epidemiology, not a broad overview of epidemiology.

If you know nothing about epidemiology, find a book on epidemiology before embarking on this book. If you know absolutely nothing about statistics, you may have a hard time with this book, even if the formal prerequisites are small.

Acknowledgements

I am grateful to my colleagues at Steno Diabetes Center Copenhagen, Dorte Vistisen and Lars Jorge Diaz, and to my long-standing collaborator and adviser Michel Hills for helpful comments and critical remarks in the development of this book.

The exposition of case-control studies relies very heavily on the one in *Statistical Models in Epidemiology* by David Clayton and Michael Hills.

Chapter 1 on simple usage of R includes parts snatched from *An Introduction to R for Epidemiology* by Martyn Plummer, Michael Hills, and Bendix Carstensen (http://bendixcarstensen.com/Epi/R-intro.pdf), developed in connection with courses over the past two decades, notably the course 'Statistical Practice in Epidemiology with R', http://bendixcarstensen.com/SPE, which has been running (almost) every summer since 2000. The Epi package has grown out of this course with major contributions by Martyn Plummer, and minor by me, Esa Läärä, and Michael Hills. I am grateful to my co-teachers at the course, Michael Hills, Lyle Gurrin, Martyn Plummer, Esa Läärä, Krista Fischer, Mark Myatt, Janne Pitkäniemi, Damien Georges, and Peter Dalgaard from whom I received much inspiration and reprimanding over the years.

My employer since 1999, Steno Diabetes Center Copenhagen, has always provided an inspiring work environment and has given me the possibility of writing this book. A special thanks goes to my colleagues in the department of Clinical Epidemiology for encouragement and daily challenges.

Copenhagen, April 2020

List of Figures

Introduction

What you should do

The code shown in each chapter is available at the website www.oup.com/companion/ carstensenEwR (this URL is case-sensitive). You will benefit from running it on your own computer and use R to look further into the various data structures you create on the way ('objects' as we call them).

Code chunks

This book is produced using `Rweave`, essentially meaning that I only ever wrote the input bits of code (shown in blue), whereas the output (what the computer replied) are as generated by R (shown in red). Occasionally, the output is omitted for want of space; another reason for you to run the code on your computer.

Some of the code chunks deserve a bit of explanation; these are given in sections starting with 'code explained:' and marked with a grey vertical bar to the left of the text. Not all code is directly epidemiology-related; there is a point in demonstrating that R has the capability to explore and display your data in ways that makes you comfortable that you have got it right. So some of the code lines merely serve to demonstrate that some data structure actually is as we claimed it would be.

I have tried to index all uses of R-functions, so you should in principle be able to use the index to find all uses of a function through the index.

Almost all of the code sections will assume that you have the `Epi` package installed, so if (when!) you get errors to the effect that some function could not be found you most likely forgot to load the `Epi` package (or some other package).

Graphs in this book

Almost all graphs in this book are produced using the base graphics package in R. The general appearance of base graphics are controlled by parameters supplied to the `par` function. The default values of these parameters are not all particularly sensible, so all graphs in this book are produced with the following setting of graphical parameters:

```
> par( mar=c(3,3,1,1), mgp=c(3,1,0)/1.6, bty="n" )
```

CODE EXPLAINED: The parameter `mar` sets the margins (measured in text lines) on the 4 sides of the plot, the 4 numbers refer to the four sides of the plot: 1: bottom, 2: left, 3: top, and 4: right. `mgp` refer to the position of 1: the axis label, 2: the labels of the tick marks, and 3: the position of the axis itself, again measured in units of lines. So setting this to `c(3,1,0)/1.6` gives values 1.875, 0.625, and 0. Finally, `bty` determines what

Epidemiology with R. Bendix Carstensen, Oxford University Press (2021). © Bendix Carstensen.
DOI: 10.1093/oso/9780198841326.003.0001

type of box, if any, is to be drawn around the graph; setting it to "n" omits a box and only leaves the axes as determined by R.

This setting of the graphical parameters for all of the graphs makes the space for the actual graph substantially larger than the default settings for the par parameters. These parameter settings are not explicitly mentioned in the code examples where graphs are produced, but they are present in all graphs.

You will find that the construction of some of the graphs are very elaborate. This is intentional; it is meant to demonstrate that you need to think carefully about all the elements of a graph in the light of the subject matter, and also that there may be features of the quantities you graph that must be reflected in the layout of a graph.

Practicing R

Occasionally you might find code where you think something like: 'Why didn't he just define the matrix so that it fitted directly to the function?' This is deliberate, because in practical circumstances you will meet data that need a bit of fidgeting before being used, and therefore need a few practical tools and tricks to get around the problems. The examples given throughout are intended to illustrate the sort of things you would normally be doing in code, including things that are not strictly on the topic of epidemiology. There is about 87.3% epidemiology and 12.7% handy tricks in this book, so do not expect a full treatise on data management in R in this book.

CHAPTER 1

Using R

The best way to learn R is to use it. Start by using it as a simple calculator, and keep on exploring what you get back by inspecting the size, shape, and content of what you create.

1.1 Installing and using R

The first thing you should do is to install R on your computer so that you can start doing simple exercises.

R is available from CRAN, the Comprehensive R Archive Network (Google it); you will find a link to installation there. If it does not work directly, it may be because your administrator has placed restrictions on what you are allowed to install on your computer.

A nice interface to R is RStudio (Google it), which is a commercial product, but RStudio has a free open source license that allows you to have a very good and handy interface to R for free, including the possibility of writing reports using Rmarkdown, Sweave, or knitr (see p. 4)

1.2 Documenting your code and results

You have probably repeatedly been told that you should comment your computer code so that you can actually remember what you intended to do with the code. And in some instances you did. If you return to un-commented code more than a fortnight after it was written you will most likely be facing the problem of reverse-engineering: trying to deduce from the code what you did (and maybe even what you intended to do). That is not always a pleasant exercise, and some people end up doing the programming from scratch again. This leaves you with a number of different programs that purportedly claim to do approximately the same. But of course never do. So the coding-first approach is a recipe for chaos in your code and results.

Therefore it is a good habit *first* in plain text to describe what you want to do, and only subsequently to write the code that does it.

It is well known that comments inside code tend to be very terse and not very easy to read, so people have come up with systems that allow you to mix proper text and code, in some contexts touted 'tools for reproducible research'. The idea is basically that you write your explanations of what you intend to do, background, etc., in a text document, and also put your R-code in the document. Then you process the document so that you get not only your original text and code, but also the results from the code in a proper text document.

Epidemiology with R. Bendix Carstensen, Oxford University Press (2021). © Bendix Carstensen.
DOI: 10.1093/oso/9780198841326.003.0002

For R the major machineries for this are `Rmarkdown` and `Sweave`/`knitr`. `Rmarkdown` as well as `Sweave` and `knitr` are systems that allow you to produce reports with text, code, results, and graphs with a single code file as input. This allows you to produce a document that accounts for every step from reading your (raw) data files to the numerical and graphical results. Moreover, your original code in conjunction with your raw data will produce the same results on any other computer. This is the essence of reproducible research; *all* decisions and choices relating to the results are embedded in the document.

It is of course only reproducible if you actually write a proper account of what you intend to do and then manage to produce code that actually does it—preferably demonstrably so. So there is indeed no such thing as a free lunch.

1.2.1 *R markdown*

You can create a skeleton `Rmarkdown` (`.rmd`) document from **RStudio** by clicking: `File→New file→R Markdown`. This will open a `Rmarkdown` document that contains a few very simple R-commands and some text.

An `Rmarkdown` document is a text file where you can put your subject-matter text describing whatever you are aiming at. The file will also contain what is called *markup* commands[1] that determine how the final document looks, such as headings, etc. More-over, and most importantly, you can insert 'chunks' of R-code, which when the document is processed will be replaced by the code *and* the results from the code. This is an important aspect of the reproducibility: any result you are quoting comes directly from the code; it has never been read and reproduced by a human (such as you or Murphy, just to mention a few).

However, this book is about *epidemiology* with R, and not an introduction to `Rmarkdown`, so you should only take this as a recommendation to learn and use `Rmarkdown` for documentation of your code and results. The specific details on the workings of `Rmarkdown` you should seek elsewhere; the Web documentation changes often, though.

1.2.2 *Sweave / knitr*

`Rweave`/`Sweave` is another markup machinery; it provides an interface to LaTeX, so you can have the full flexibility of this with detailed control of the look of your document. This book is produced using `Rweave`. If you intend to maintain larger documents such as multi-chapter reports (or a book!), and in particular if more than one person is to work on it, this is the set of tools you must learn. But not from this book.

An amended version of `Rweave` is `knitr` that provides extended facilities for the code and results chunks such as syntax-coloured code. These tools are only mentioned here for the sake of completeness, no further treatise is offered in the book.

1.2.3 *Coding style in R*

Different people have different coding styles; that is how they place variable name, parentheses, and operators relative to each other. There is no particular reason that you

---

[1] In the olden days when journalists were typing their manuscripts on physical paper, the typesetters needed instructions as how to typeset the text, i.e. what should be headings, what should be in italics, etc. This information was added to the typed manuscripts by hand using a special set of symbols and markings, called the *markup*. The name `Rmarkdown` is a pun on this. You may also know that HTML is an abbreviation of '**h**yper**t**ext **m**arkup **l**anguage', since it describes how to display text (and other information) on your screen.

should take over precisely the coding style I am (trying to be) using in this book; many will disagree to some or all of my points. But you should give it a good thought because you can make your code more readable.

I have largely adhered to the following general rules in the code you see in this book, mainly for the sake of readability:

- Put spaces around the assignment operator ('`<-`')
- Let any comma be followed by a space.
- Put spaces around all operators such as `+`, `/`, etc., except around '`:`'
- Use fairly short and meaningful names for variables and objects. Very long object names makes it difficult to get the meaning of the code (and increases the likelihood of typos). This is one of the most difficult tasks in programming, but it pays to spend time on it. `long_name_proponents` do exist, though.
- Use short lines of code; a command can be broken across several line at (almost) any point. Normally it is done after a comma.
- Occasionally you may want to put more than one statement on the same line. That can be done by separating statements with a semi colon (;).
- When using braces ('`{ }`') let the opening and closing braces be at the same position on the line. Putting them each on a separate line is sometimes useful. The closing brace should always be on a line of its own.
- When putting the arguments of a function on separate lines, place all arguments indented at the opening bracket of the function.
- When calling functions with many arguments, it is sometimes useful to make the equal signs between argument names and argument values vertically aligned (this is in conflict with the previous point).

Finally, keep in mind that when writing a piece of R-code it is only a *secondary* purpose to get the data processing and calculations correct; the *primary* purpose of the code is to document that what you claim to have done is actually what you did do.

1.2.4 *R lingo*

When talking about R, a few words and phrases are used frequently:

gets the official pronunciation of the assignment operator '`<-`'

of the official pronunciation of using a function on a argument, 'f of x' meaning `f(x)`. So whenever you hear 'glm of ...' you should type `glm( )` and wait for what goes in between the brackets.

console the window in RStudio where the results are displayed and where you can type the occasional command you do not wish inserted in your document.

script window the window in RStudio where you type your code (or `Rmarkdown` code and text)

arguments what is supplied to functions inside brackets. Each argument has a *name* which is placed to the left of an '`=`', and a *value* which is placed to the right of it. So `name=value`. The argument names are characteristics of the function; you supply the values. These pairs are separated by commas.

coerce forcing one type of object to become an object of a different type. For example: the function `as.numeric` coerces its argument to mode numeric. It will, for example, transform the character "7" to the number 7, and the character string "seven" to missing, NA.

class what class an object is. The class of an object determines how functions like summary, plot, etc. behave when an object of a given class is supplied as the first argument to the function.

mode what type of element the object consists of; see ?mode.

wrapper a function that calls another function with a set of (often used) prespecified values for some of the arguments.

package a collection of functions (and/or datasets) that can be attached to your R-session so that you have access to the functions. Epi is one such package. Oddly, a package is attached (loaded) for use by the function library().

1.3 Simple usage of R

The following (as any other piece of code you meet in this book) is intended for you to try out and also change a bit to get further insight about the objects you are manipulating. It introduces a number of basic features of R that are best demonstrated if you explore them yourself. Therefore, only some of the results of the code are shown; you only get to see the missing ones by running R yourself.

When you start R you will see a '>' at the beginning of the line in the console. When you type code in there (or transfer it from the script using CTRL-ENTER) R will know whether you have typed a complete expression. If you have, you will see the result of it (if any is produced), but if you have not completed the command, the next line will have a + at the beginning, indicating that R expects more to come.

1.3.1 Using R as a calculator

Typing 2+2 will return the answer 4, typing 2^3 will return the answer 8 (2 to the power of 3), typing log(10) will return the natural logarithm of 10, which is 2.3026, and typing sqrt(25) will return the square root of 25.

Instead of printing the result you can store it in an *object*, say

```
> a <- 2+2
```

and you can actually also do

```
> 2+2 -> a
```

The contents of the object a can be printed by typing a. Try that.

1.3.2 A functional language

R is a *functional* language; everything you ever do is to call a function that transforms something to something else and possibly assigns it or just prints it; try for example:

```
> x <- 1:10
> x
```

There does not seem to be any functions here? The first statement actually uses the function ':', which takes two arguments, in this case 1 and 10, and returns a sequence of numbers with distance 1 and assigns it to x (you can actually write `":"(1,10)` if you wish). The second statement implicitly invokes the `print` function to print the vector x. Using a function on x without assigning it will automatically invoke the print function and print it on your screen (console).

From a practical point of view what you are doing is creating a vector of the numbers 1 to 10 and storing it in a so-called *object* called x, so you can access it later; for example, printing it just by typing its name, as above.

A couple of simple functions are

```
> sum(x)
> sd(x)
> diff(x)
> cumsum(x)
> rev(x)
> prod(x)
> x > 7
> x >= 7
```

Try them and find out what they do.

Probability functions

Standard probability functions are readily available in R. For example, the probability below 1.96 in a standard normal (i.e. Gaussian) distribution is obtained with

```
> pnorm(1.96)
```

while

```
> pchisq(3.84,1)
```

will return the probability below 3.84 in a χ^2 distribution on 1 degree of freedom, and

```
> pchisq(3.84,1,lower.tail=FALSE)
```

will return the probability above 3.84.

Exercises

1. Calculate $\sqrt{3^2 + 4^2}$.
2. Find the probability above 4.3 in a chi-squared distribution on 1 degree of freedom.

Objects and functions

All commands in R are *functions* which act on *objects*. One important kind of object is a *vector*, which is an ordered collection of numbers, or an ordered collection of character strings. Examples of vectors are (4, 6, 1, 2.2), which is a numeric vector with 4 components, and ('Charles Darwin', 'Alfred Wallace') which is a vector of character strings with 2 components. The components of a vector must be of the same type (numeric, character, or logical). The combine function `c()`, together with the assignment operator, is used to create vectors. Thus

```
> v <- c(4, 6, 1, 2.2)
```

creates a vector v with components 4, 6, 1, 2.2 by first combining the 4 numbers 4, 6, 1, 2.2 in order and then assigning the result to the vector v.

Collections of components of different types are called *lists*, and are created with the
`list()` function. Thus

```
> m <- list(4:7, six=6, "name of company")
> m
[[1]]
[1]  4  5  6  7

$six
[1]  6

[[3]]
[1] "name of company"
```

creates a `list` with 3 components. `lists` allows elements of different kinds, in this case
two numeric vectors (leenth 4 an 1) and a character vector; and in this case the second
element is named.

The main differences between the numbers 4, 6, 1, 2.2 and the vector `v` is that along
with `v` is stored information about what sort of object it is and hence how it is printed
and how it is combined with other objects. Try

```
> v
> 3+v
> 3*v
```

and you will see that R understands what to do in each case. This may seem trivial, but
remember that unlike most statistical packages there are many different kinds of object
in R.

You can get a description of the structure of any object using the function `str()`. For
example, `str(v)` shows that `v` is numeric with 4 components.

What makes R different: functions

R also gives you the possibility of writing your own functions; they need not be very fancy,
nor do they need to have any arguments. In this book we will frequenty use probabilities
π and *odds*, $\omega = \pi/(1-\pi)$, so we will want to be able to convert easily from one to another.
This can be done by defining functions for the conversions:

```
> p2o <- function(p) p/(1-p)
> o2p <- function(o) o/(1+o)
```

These functions will convert between probabilities and odds:

```
> p2o(0.25)
> o2p(8)
```

What do you think you get if you write `o2p( p2o(0.25) )`?

A function in R is defined by `function` and the value returned by the function is the
value of the *last* statement. To make it a bit more clear how a function is defined we could
have written

```
> p2o <-
+ function( p )
+   {
+   odds <-  p / ( 1 - p )
+   odds
+   }
```

The function is defined by naming the *arguments* (what is between the ()s—in this case one, p), and then defining what is to be computed from these in the *body* of the function (what is between the {}s). The *value* of the function when called with appropriate argument(s) is the value of the last expession in the function body, in this case just 'odds'.

1.3.3 *Sequences*

It is not always necessary to type out all the components of a vector to create one. For example, the vector (15,20,25,...,85) can be created with

```
> seq(15, 85, by=5)
```

and the vector (5,20,25,...,85) can be created with

```
> c(5,seq(20, 85, by=5))
```

It is also possible to repeat vectors in complex patterns; try

```
> rep( c(3,2,7), c(1,4,3) )
> rep( c(3,2,7), 5 )
> rep( c(3,2,7), each=5 )
```

A particularly simple form of a sequence is one where the step length is 1; this is created by ':'

```
> 7:10
> 8:3.5
> 3.7:8.1
```

You can learn more about a function by typing '?' followed by the function name. For example, ?seq gives information about the syntax and usage of the function seq().

Exercises

1. Create a vector w with components $1, -1, 2, -2$
2. Print this vector (to the screen)
3. Obtain a description of w using str()
4. Create the vector w+1, and print it.
5. Create the vector (0, 1, 5, 10, 15, ... , 75) using c() and seq().
6. Create a vector with 20 elements equally spaced between 7 and 23

1.3.4 *The births data*

The most important example of a vector in epidemiology is the data on a variable recorded for a group of subjects. A collection of these can be put side by side to form a dataset, in R called a data.frame. As an example we shall use the births data which concern 500 mothers who had singleton births in a large London hospital. These data are available as an R data.frame called births in the Epi package, with the variable shown in Table 1.1. The easiest way to access the births data is first to load the Epi package with

```
> library(Epi)
```

and then to load the data with

```
> data(births)
```

Table 1.1 *Variables in the births data frame*

Variable	Units or Coding	Type	Name
Person id	–	categorical	`id`
Birth weight	grams	metric	`bweight`
Birth weight < 2500 g	1=yes, 0=no	categorical	`lowbw`
Gestational age	weeks	metric	`gestwks`
Gestational age < 37 weeks	1=yes, 0=no	categorical	`preterm`
Maternal age	years	metric	`matage`
Maternal hypertension	1=hypertensive, 0=normal	categorical	`hyp`
Sex of baby	1=male, 2=female	categorical	`sex`

You get an overview from the `Epi` package documentation by

```
> ?births
```

Some of the variables which make up these data take integer values while others are numeric taking measurements as values. For most variables the integer values are just codes for different categories, such as `"male"` and `"female"`, which are coded 1 and 2 for the variable `sex`.

The function

```
> str(births)
```

shows that the object `births` is a data frame with 500 observations of 8 variables. The names and types of the variables are also shown together with the first couple of values of each variable.

Exercises

1. The data frame `diet` in the `Epi` package contains data from a follow-up study with coronary heart disease as the end-point. Load these data with

   ```
   > data(diet)
   ```

   and print the contents of the data frame to the screen.
2. Check that you now have two objects, `births` and `diet`, in your work space, using `ls()` or the `lls()` from `Epi`.
3. Obtain a description of the object `diet`.
4. Remove the object `diet` with the command

   ```
   > rm(diet)
   ```

   Check that you only have the object `births` left in your workspace.

1.3.5 *Referencing parts of a data frame*

Typing `births` will list the entire data frame—not usually very helpful. Now try

```
> births[1,"bweight"]
```

This will list the value taken by the first subject for the `bweight` variable. Similarly

```
> births[2,"bweight"]
```

will list the value taken by the second subject for bweight, and so on. To list the data for the first 10 persons for the bweight variable, try

```
> births[1:10, "bweight"]
```

and to list all the data for this variable, try

```
> births[, "bweight"]
```

An alternative way of referring to a variable in a data frame is using the '$'

```
> births$bweight
```

Exercises

1. Print the data on the variable gestwks for subject 7 in the births data frame.
2. Print all the data for subject 7.
3. Print all the data on the variable gestwks.

1.3.6 *Summaries*

A good way to start an analysis is to ask for a summary of the data by typing

```
> summary(births)
```

To see just the names of the variables in the data frame try

```
> names(births)
```

A bit more information is obtained by

```
> str(births)
```

Variables in a data frame can be referred to by name, but to do so it is necessary also to specify the name of the data frame. Thus births$hyp refers to the variable hyp in the births data frame, and typing births$hyp will print the data on this variable. To summarize the variable hyp try

```
> summary(births$hyp)
```

So you see that summary behaves differently when you supply a data frame and vector to it.

In most datasets there will be some missing values. The summary shows the number of missing values for each variable, indicated by NA (Not Available).

The summary is a *generic* function, which means that many clsses of R objects will have summary methods defined, for example summary.lm, which will give a summary of a linear model. So summary will work with many different types of R objects, behaving differently according to the type of object.

1.3.7 *Generating new variables*

New variables can be produced using assignment together with the usual mathematical operations and functions:

```
    +      -      *      /      ^      sqrt      log      exp
```

The sign ^ means 'to the power of', sqrt (x) means 'square root of *x*', $\sqrt{x}$, and log means 'natural logarithm'. An extensive discussion on the use of logarithms in statistical analysis is in section 4.8.1 on p. 87.

The transform function allows you to transform or generate variables in a data frame. For example, try

```
> births <- transform( births,
+                            num1 = 1,
+                            logbw = log( bweight ),
+                             avg = bweight / gestwks )
```

The variable logbw is the natural logarithm of birth weight, and avg is the birth weight per gestational week.

dplyr

The package dplyr provides a slightly different syntax for the same using the pipe operator %>% to indicate that first we have births, and then we subject it to a mutation:

```
> library( dplyr )
> bth <- births %>% mutate( num1 = 1,
+                           logbw = log( bweight ),
+                            avg = bweight / gestwks )
```

More logically, we might put the assignment of the result at the end to indicate that the assignment comes after the mutation:

```
> births %>% mutate( num1 = 1,
+                    logbw = log( bweight ),
+                     avg = bweight / gestwks ) -> bth
```

All three sets of code will produce the same result, namely the births data frame with three extra variables. The mutate function is, however, more versatile; for example, it allows further calculations on variables defined inside mutate, which transform does not.

The package dplyr comes with a large set of functions for data frame manipulation, but as this is a book on epidemiology we shall not venture further into this.

1.3.8 *Logical variables*

Logical variables take the values TRUE or FALSE, and behave mostly like factors. New variables can be created which are logical functions of existing variables. For example

```
> low <- births$bweight < 2000
> str( low )
```

creates a logical variable low with levels TRUE and FALSE, according to whether bweight is less than 2000 or not. The logical expressions which R allow are

$$! \qquad == \qquad < \qquad <= \qquad > \qquad >= \qquad !=$$

The first is logical negation, the second equals, and the last is logical *not* equals. One common use of logical variables is to restrict a command to a subset of the data. For example, to list the values taken by bweight for hypertensive women, try

```
> births$bweight [births$hyp==1]
```

If you want the entire data frame restricted to hypertensive women try

```
> births [births$hyp==1,]
```

The `subset ()` function allows you to take a subset of a data frame. Try

```
> subset (births, hyp==1)
```

You can check whether birth weight is smaller than 2500 grams among the first 10 births:

```
> births$bweight [1:10] < 3000
 [1]   TRUE FALSE   TRUE FALSE FALSE FALSE FALSE FALSE FALSE FALSE
```

and you can also find out where the TRUE values are:

```
> which ( births$bweight [1:10] < 3000 )
[1] 1 3
```

Caveat: You cannot use TRUE or FALSE as names of variables. But you can abbreviate TRUE and FALSE as T and F, and you *can* use T and F as variable names. If you do, you can get almost impentrable errors or, even worse, undetected misbeaviour, some very hard to find. So: never call a variable T or F, and always use the full form TRUE and FALSE.

Exercises

1. Create a logical variable called `early` according to whether `gestwks` is less than 30 or not. Make a frequency table of `early` using `table`.
2. Print the `id` numbers of women with `gestwks` less than 30 weeks.

1.3.9 *Turning a variable into a factor*

In R categorical variables are known as *factors*, and the different categories are called the *levels* of the factor. Variables such as `hyp` and `sex` are originally coded using integer codes, and by default R will interpret these codes as numeric values taken by the variables. But we would never want to do calculations on these numerical values; they would only ever be used to indicate a category.

For R to recognize that the codes refer to categories it is necessary to convert the variables to factors, and in order to make code and results human readable it is also necessary to label the levels. To convert the variable `hyp` to a factor, try

```
> hyp <- factor ( births$hyp )
> lls ()
```

The latter shows that `hyp` is both in your work space (as a factor) and in the `births` data frame (as a numeric variable). It is better to use the `transform` function on the data frame, so that the `hyp` variable in the data frame is converted to a factor:

```
> births <- transform ( births, hyp=factor (hyp) )
> str ( births )
'data.frame':        500 obs.  of   11 variables:
 $ id      : num  1 2 3 4 5 6 7 8 9 10 ...
 $ bweight: num   2974 3270 2620 3751 3200 ...
 $ lowbw  : num   0 0 0 0 0 0 0 0 0 ...
 $ gestwks: num   38.5 NA 38.2 39.8 38.9 ...
 $ preterm: num   0 NA 0 0 0 0 0 0 0 ...
```

```
$ matage : num   34 30 35 31 33 33 29 37 36 39 ...
$ hyp     : Factor w/ 2 levels "0","1": 1 1 1 2 1 1 1 1 1 ...
$ sex     : num   2 1 2 1 1 2 2 1 2 1 ...
$ num1    : num   1 1 1 1 1 1 1 1 1 1 ...
$ logbw   : num   8 8.09 7.87 8.23 8.07 ...
$ avg     : num   77.2 NA 68.7 94.2 82.3 ...
```

which shows that hyp, in the births data frame, is now a factor with two levels, labelled
'0' and '1'—the original values taken by the variable. It is better to assign labels as (say)
"normal" and "hyper" with

```
> births <- transform( births,
+                      hyp = factor(hyp,labels=c("normal","hyper")) )
> str(births$hyp)
```

You may want a different order than the numerical defaults of the levels; one way of
achieveing this is using the levels argument:

```
> births <- transform( births,
+                      early = factor( preterm,
+                                      levels=c(1,0),
+                                      labels=c("Pre","Norm")) )
> with( births, table( preterm, early ) )
```

The naming of the arguments is a bit odd; levels refer to the *in*coming values (of
preterm) and labels to the *out*going values (in early). However, if afterwards you want
to know what values the factor assumes, we refer to these as the levels of the factor:

```
> levels( births$early)
```

Internally, the factor levels are stored as the integers 1,2,..., and the (names of the) levels
of the factor in a separate structure. That way the names of the levels are only stored once,
saving space.

Manipulating factor levels

When producing tables you may want to have levels of a factor in a specfic order or even
combine some of the levels. Using the dataset diet, try

```
> data( diet )
> table( diet$job )
    Driver   Conductor Bank worker
       102          84         151
> table( relevel(diet$job,2) )
  Conductor      Driver Bank worker
         84         102         151
> table( relevel(diet$job,"Bank worker") )
Bank worker      Driver   Conductor
        151         102          84
> table( Relevel(diet$job,3:1) )
Bank worker   Conductor      Driver
        151          84         102
> table( Relevel(diet$job,list(3,1:2)) )
    Bank worker Driver+Conductor
            151              186
```

The base R function `relevel` (lower case) only has the capability of moving a specific level of the factor up as the first—a facility which is handy in regression modelling. The Epi function `Relevel` (capilatized) allows combination of factor levels too.

   `Relevel` also allows grouping via a look-up in a table—try

```
> example (Relevel)
```

to see examples of this.

   If you take a subset of a data frame, you may end up with a factor that has a level that is not assumed:

```
> subdiet <- subset ( diet, job!="Driver" )
> table ( subdiet$job )
```

In some contexts this may be impractical; the way to get rid of the non-used levels is by using `factor`:

```
> table ( factor (subdiet$job) )
```

Exercises

1. In the `births` data frame, convert the variable `sex` into a factor.
2. Label the levels of `sex` as `"M"` and `"W"`.
3. In the `diet` dataset, combine levels `Driver` and `Conductor` to a level called `Bus employee`.

Grouping values of a quantitative variable

For a numeric variable like `matage` it is occasionally useful to group the values and to create a new factor representing the grouping. This should only be used for exploration of data; modelling effects of a quantitative variable should *never* be based on a grouping (see Chapter 9, p. 219).

   For example we might cut the values taken by `matage` into the groups 20–29, 30–34, 35–39, 40–44, and then create a factor called `agegrp` with 4 levels corresponding to the four groups. The best way of doing this is with the function `cut`:

```
> births <- transform ( births, agegrp = cut (matage,
+                                     breaks = c(25,30,35,40,45),
+                                     right = FALSE) )
> table ( births$agegrp, exclude=NULL )

[25,30) [30,35) [35,40) [40,45)    <NA>
     68     200     194      36       2
```

> CODE EXPLAINED: `transform` is used to define a new variable (a factor), `agegrp`, in the `births` data frame. The argument `right` is a logical indicating whether the right end-point should be included in each interval; we want the left end-point to be included, so we set it to `FALSE`. Persons with a value of `matage` less than 25 or larger than 45 will be transformed to `NA`. `table` will ignore `NA`s, unless instructed to include everything by `exclude=NULL`.

By default the factor levels are labelled [20-25), [25-30), etc., where [20-25) refers to the interval which includes the left end (20) but not the right end (25). This was brought about by using the argument `right=FALSE`. When `right=TRUE` (which is the default) the intervals include the right end but not the left.

It is important to realize that observations which are not inside the range specified in the `breaks()` part of the command result in missing values for the new factor. For example

```
> births <- transform( births, agegrp=cut(matage,
+                                          breaks=c(20,30,35),
+                                          right=FALSE) )
> summary(births$agegrp)
```

Only observations from 20 up to, but not including 35, are included. For the rest, `agegrp` is coded missing. This will not immediately show up if you use `table`, but the argument `exclude=NULL` will remedy this; try

```
> table( births$agegrp )
> table( births$agegrp, exclude=NULL )
> addmargins( table( births$agegrp, exclude=NULL ) )
```

`addmargins` adds margins to any type of a table; it can be any type of margins, not only sums (which is the default).

You can specify that you want to cut a variable into a given number of intervals of equal length by specifying the number of intervals. For example

```
> births <- transform( births, agegrp=cut(matage,
+                                          breaks=5,
+                                          right=FALSE) )
> table( births$agegrp )
[23,27) [27,31) [31,35) [35,39) [39,43)
     16      83     171     166      64
```

shows 5 intervals of width 4 years, spanning the range of `matage`. This is rarely useful, and almost certainly irrelevant w.r.t. generalizability, because the grouping depends on the distribution of the variable in the particular study population.

This, however, is only one of the many pitfalls in grouping data; see Chapter 9.

Exercises

1. Summarize the numeric variable `gestwks`, which records the length of gestation for the baby, and make a note of the range of values.
2. Create a new factor `gest4` which cuts `gestwks` at 20, 35, 37, 39, and 45 weeks, including the left-hand end, but not the right-hand. Make a table of the frequencies for the four levels of `gest4`.
3. Create a new factor `gest5` which cuts `gestwks` into 5 equal intervals, and make a table of frequencies.

1.3.10 *Tables*

When starting to look at any new data frame the first step is to check that the values of the variables make sense and correspond to the codes defined in the coding schedule. For categorical variables (factors) this can be done by looking at one-way frequency tables and checking that only the specified codes (levels) occur. A very useful function for making tables is `stat.table` from the `Epi` package.

The distribution of the factors `hyp` and `sex` can be viewed by typing

```
> data( births )
> stat.table( hyp, data=births )
> stat.table( sex, data=births )
```

Their cross-tabulation is obtained by typing

```
> stat.table( list(hyp,sex), data=births )
 ---------------------
      -------sex-------
 hyp        1       2
 ---------------------
 0        221     207
 1         43      29
 ---------------------
```

Cross-tabulations are useful when checking for consistency, but because no distinction is drawn between the response variable and any explanatory variables, they are not necessarily useful as a way of presenting data, and as you see, rather meaningless if the variables you tabulate are not properly labelled factors.

Tables of means and other things

To obtain the mean of bweight by sex, try

```
> stat.table(sex, mean(bweight), data=births)
```

The headings of the table can be improved with

```
> stat.table( sex,
+             list("Mean birth weight"=mean(bweight)),
+             data=births )
```

To make a two-way table of mean birth weight by sex and hypertension, first convert sex and hyp to factors for readability:

```
> births <- transform( births, sex = factor(sex, labels=c("M","W")),
+                              hyp = factor(hyp, labels=c("No","Yes")) )
> stat.table( list(sex, hyp),
+             mean(bweight),
+             margins = TRUE,
+               data = births )
```

and to tabulate the count as well as the mean, including the margins:

```
> stat.table( list(sex,hyp),
+             list(count(),
+                  mean(bweight)),
+             margins=TRUE,
+             data=births )
```

Available functions for the cells of the table are count, mean, weighted.mean, sum, min, max, quantile, median, IQR, and ratio. The last of these is useful for rates and odds. For example, to make a table of the odds of low birth weight by hypertension, try

```
> stat.table( hyp,
+             list("odds"=ratio(lowbw,1-lowbw,100)),
+             data=births)
```

The scale factor 100 makes the odds per 100, so essentially %. Margins can be added to the tables, as required. For example, you will do

```
> stat.table(sex,
+            mean(bweight),
+            margins = TRUE,
+               data = births )
```

for a one-way table. For a two-way table, you can try

```
> stat.table( list(sex,hyp),
+             mean(bweight),
+            margins = c(TRUE,FALSE),
+                data = births )
> stat.table( list(sex,hyp),
+             mean(bweight),
+            margins = TRUE,
+                data = births )
```

Exercises

1. Make a table of median birth weight by `sex`.
2. Do the same for gestation time, but include `count` as a function to be tabulated along with `median`. Note that when there are missing values for the variable being summarized the count refers to the number of non-missing observations for the row variable, not the summarized variable.
3. Create a table showing the mean gestation time for the baby by `hyp` and `lowbw`, together with margins for both.
4. Make a table showing the odds of hypertension by sex of the baby.

1.3.11 *Reading data*

R can read data from many different formats; the functions for reading various data formats are found in a number of different packages. So remember to read the documentation; there are many pitfalls, and since this book is not about data no comprehensive overview is given here. Reading data without reading the documentation of the function you use to read data is a prescription of erroneous data.

When reading data, a number of points should be kept in mind that may give rise to funny data if forgotten:

- Variable names—are they in the first line of the data file?
- How are missing values coded?
- How are categorical variables (factors) coded?
- How are dates represented?
- What is the decimal separator?

Different function for reading data will handle these issues differently, and most will have a large number of arguments that control how data are read.

The following functions will cover many needs you may have:

- Plain files with spaces separating variables: use `read.table`, for example:

```
> fem <- read.table( "http://bendixcarstensen.com/SPE/data/fem.dat",
+                    header = TRUE,
+               na.strings = c("-99","NA") )
```

As you see, R will recognize a URL and read directly from it. In the file, the first line contains the variable names, and missing values are represented either by -99 or NA.

- Comma-separated files: .csv, use the function read.csv or read.csv2 depending on whether the file is with comma or semicolon as separator.
- Clipboard: a quick and dirty way to get in a small chunk of data is to highlight the data on your screen (e.g. in Excel) and press CTRL-C ('copy'). The data is then placed on your clipboard. You can then just do

```
> qad <- read.table( "clipboard" )
```

—but you will still have the all the issues with missing data representation, etc.

- Data from other statistical packages such as SAS or Stata: use the functionalities in the haven package:

```
> help( package = haven )
```

The package haven also contains facilities to *write* data in formats for other statistics pages.

- Excel files: use the package xlsx, see help(package = xlsx) to obtain more information.
- SQL databases: use the package RODBC, see help(package = RODBC) to obtain more information.

1.3.12 *Saving data*

Saving the work space

When exiting from R you are offered the chance of saving all the objects in your current work space. If you do so, the work space is re-instated next time you start R. It is only occasionally useful to do this. However, if you choose to do so it is worth tidying things up, because the work space can fill up with temporary objects, and it is easy to forget what these are when you resume the session.

The general advice is *not* to save the workspace.

Saving R objects in a file

The command read.table() is relatively slow because it carries out quite a lot of processing as it reads the data. To avoid doing this more than once you can save the data frame, which includes the R information, and read from this saved file in future. For example,

```
> save(births, file = "births.Rda")
```

will save the births data frame in the file births.Rda. By default the data frame is saved as a binary file, but the option ascii=TRUE can be used to save it as a text file. You can save more than one object in an R-file, they need not be data frames, and they can be fitted models. For example

```
> save(births, p2o, o2p, file = "births.Rda")
```

To load the object(s) from an .Rda file, use

```
> load("births.Rda", verbose=TRUE)
```

The commands `save()` and `load()` can be used with any R objects, but they are particularly useful when dealing with large data frames. The `verbose` argument lists the names of the objects loaded.

1.3.13 *The search path*

R organizes objects in different positions on a search path. The command

```
> search()
```

shows these positions. The first is the work space, or global environment; the next ones are packages attached by `library`. To see what is in the work space try

```
> objects()
> ls()
> lls()
```

To see what is in the Epi package, try

```
> objects("package:Epi")
```

When you type the name of an object, R looks for it in the order of the search path and will return the first object with this name that it finds. This is why it is best to start your session with a clean workspace; otherwise, you might have an object in your workspace from an old session that masks one later in the search path.

Attaching a data frame

The function `objects(1)` shows the objects in the workspace. To refer to variables in the `births` data frame by name it is necessary to specify the name of the data frame, as in `births$hyp`. This is quite cumbersome, and provided you are working primarily with one data frame, it can help to put a copy of the variables from a data frame in their own position on the search path. This is done with the function `attach`:

```
> attach(births)
```

which places a copy of the variables in the `births` data frame in position 2. You can verify this with

```
> objects(2)
```

which shows the objects in this position are the variables from the `births` data frame. Note that the packages have now been moved up one position, as shown by the `search()` function.

When you type the command

```
> hyp
```

R will look in the first position where it fails to find `hyp`, then the second position where it finds `hyp` (namely as a column in `births`), which now gets printed.

Although convenient, attaching a data frame can give rise to confusion, quite a lot actually. For example, when you create a new object from the variables in an attached data frame, as in

```
> subgrp <- bweight[hyp==1]
```

the object subgrp will be in your workspace (position 1 on the search path), not in position 2. To demonstrate this, try (ls is another name for the function objects)

```
> ls(1)
> ls(2)
```

Similarly, if you modify the data frame in the workspace the changes will not carry through to the attached version of the data frame. The best advice is to regard any operation on an attached data frame as temporary, intended only to produce output such as summaries and tabulations.

Beware of attaching a data frame more than once—the second attached copy will be attached in position 2 of the search path, while the first copy will be moved up to position 3. You can see this with

```
> attach(births)
> search()
```

Having several copies of the same dataset can lead to great confusion. To detach a data frame, use the command

```
> detach(births)
```

which will detach the copy in position 2 and move everything else down one position. To detach the second copy, repeat the command detach(births).

Using with

The main purpose of attaching a data frame is to avoid typing births$ in front of every variable name used. Another way of avoiding this is to wrap the expressions in with, such as

```
> with( births, plot( gestwks, bweight ) )
```

The first argument is a data frame; the second argument is an expression where variable names are assumed to come from the data frame. You can use other variable names too; they will be taken from the global environment.

Exercises

1. Use search() to make sure you have no data frames attached.
2. Use objects(1) to check that you have the data frame births in your work space.
3. Verify that typing births$hyp will print the data on the variable hyp but typing hyp will not.
4. Attach the births data frame in position 2 and check that the variables from this data frame are now in position 2.
5. Verify that typing hyp will now print the data on the the variable hyp.
6. Summarize the variable bweight for hypertensive women.

1.4 Graphics

There are two main graphics systems used in R: base graphics, which is an integral part of any R distribution, and ggplot2 (gg referring to grammar of graphics), which is a separate package that you need to install, which has a different syntax, and which is not compatible with base graphics. ggplot2 is part of the tidyverse packages.

Besides these two there is also `lattice` graphics that allow quite elaborate graphs of multidimensional structures, however, at the price of quite a complicated interface. In this book we will mainly be using base graphics, though.

1.4.1 *ggplot2*

The grammar of graphics underlies the package `ggplot2`, which defines graphs as graphical objects (`grobs`) that can be modified by adding different aspects of the graph such as themes.

It is not as easy to master as base graphics, but the graphs (particular multiframe displays) will be more consistent. However, this graphical system is an entire (large) topic of its own, and will not be treated in any detail in this book; a few examples of its use will be shown though. The `ggplot2` package is part of the `tidyverse` environment; see Chapter 1.9, p. 39.

1.4.2 *Base graphics*

The plotting model of base graphics is emulating your pencil (or fountain pen): ink on paper. Each command in base graphics puts something on the graph, and you cannot remove it. If you get it wrong, you will have to start over—which is not so bad. You just run the code again, that is, unless you are typing along in the console window—in which case, do not do that.

If you just issue plot commnds, the graph will appear on the screen; if you want to put the graph in a particular file, you must open a graphics *device* before the plotting commnds, and close it afterwards. For example, if you want a plot in a `pdf` file you will open the `pdf` device using `pdf()` and close it using `dev.off()`:

```
> pdf( "a_graph.pdf" )
> x <- seq(1,5,0.01)
> plot( x, (x-2)*(x-4) )
> dev.off()
```

This will create the file `a_graph.pdf` in your current directory (if you do not know which that is, use `getwd()`)

You can get a list of available devices by

```
> ?Devices
```

(must be a capital `D`).

1.4.3 *Simple base graphs*

There are three kinds of plotting functions in base graphics:

1. Functions that generate a new plot, e.g. `hist()` and `plot()`.
2. Functions that add extra things to an existing plot, e.g. `lines()` and `text()`.
3. Functions that allow you to interact with the plot, e.g. `locator()` and `identify()`.

The normal procedure for making a graph in R is to make a fairly simple initial plot and then add on points, lines, text, etc., preferably in a script.

Plot on the screen

Load the births data and get an overview of the variables:

```
> library(Epi)
> data( births )
```

Now attach the data frame and look at the birth-weight distribution with

```
> attach(births)
> hist(bweight)
```

The histogram can be refined—take a look at the possible options with

```
> ?hist
```

and try some of the options, for example

```
> hist(bweight, col="gray", border="white")
```

To look at the relationship between birth weight and gestational weeks, try

```
> plot(gestwks, bweight)
```

You can change the plot symbol by the option pch=. If you want to see all the plot symbols, try

```
> plot(1:25, pch=1:25)
```

or, using the rep function to generate a grid of points,

```
> plot( rep(1:5,5), rep(1:5,each=5), pch=1:25,
+       cex=5, xlim=c(0,6), ylim=c(0,6), lwd=4 )
> text( rep(1:5,5)+0.3, rep(1:5,each=5), 1:25 )
```

Sometimes the default graph window in RStudio is too small to hold your graph. You can open another graph window outside of RStudio by

```
> RStudioGD()
```

(RStudioGraphicsDevice). Your graphs will then go there and you can just swap to this the usual way (using Alt-Tab, i.e. holding down the Alt key and repeatedly pressing the Tab key, and releasing the Alt once you have found your graph window).

Exercises

1. Make a plot of the birth weight versus maternal age with

```
> plot(matage, bweight)
```

2. Label the axes with

```
> plot(matage, bweight, xlab="Maternal age", ylab="Birth weight (g)")
```

Colours

There are many colours recognized by R. You can list them all by colours() or, equivalently, colors() (R allows you to use British or American spelling). To colour the points of birth weight versus gestational weeks, try

```
> plot(gestwks, bweight, pch=16, col="green")
```

This creates a solid mass of colour in the centre of the cluster of points and it is no longer possible to see individual points. You can recover this information by overwriting the points with black circles using the `points()` function:

```
> points(gestwks, bweight)
```

R has functions that generate vectors of colours for you. For example,

```
> rainbow(4)
```

produces a vector with 4 colours (not immediately human readable, though). There other functions that generates other sequences of colours, type `?rainbow` to see them.

Grey tones are produced by the function `gray` (or `grey`), which takes a numerical argument between 0 and 1; `gray(0)` is black and `gray(1)` is white. Try

```
> plot( 0:10, pch=16, cex=3, col=gray(0:10/10) )
> points( 0:10, pch=1, cex=3 )
```

Colours can be given explicitly in the RGB-space (red, green, blue) as a character string `"#RRGGBB"` where R, G, and B are hexadecimal[2] digits (0–9,A–F).

There is a number of functions in base R to manipulate colours; try, for example,

```
> col2rgb("orange")
> rgb(t(col2rgb("orange")),m=256)
```

There is also the possibility of generating semi-transparent colours, using for example `adjustcolor`. This is used in the function `matshade` that plots confidence bands as shaded areas.

Some thought has been put into constructing functions that generate sequences of colours useful in more advanced graphs; two such packages are `RColorBrewer` and `viridis`. It is left to you to explore these further; try, for example,

```
> help(package = RColorBrewer)
```

Adding to a plot

As we just saw, `points()` is one of several functions that *add* elements to an existing plot. By using these functions, you can create quite complex graphs in small steps.

Suppose we wish to recreate the plot of birth weight versus gestational weeks using different colours for male and female babies. To start with an empty plot, try

```
> attach( births )
> plot( gestwks, bweight, type="n" )
```

Even if nothing is plotted, the axes are constructed so that all points will be contained in the plot.

Then we can add the points with the `points` function:

```
> points( gestwks[sex==1], bweight[sex==1], col="blue" )
> points( gestwks[sex==2], bweight[sex==2], col="red"  )
```

---

[2] Refers to the base 16 representation of numbers using digits 0–9,A–F, with A represnting 10, F representing 15, and, say, 1B representing 16+11=27. A two-digit hexadecimal number can represent the numbers from 0 through 255 ($16^2 - 1$).

To add a legend explaining the colours, try

```
> legend( "topleft", pch=1,
+          legend = c("Boys","Girls"),
+             col = c("blue","red"   ) )
```

This should put the legend in the top left-hand corner.

Finally, we can add a title to the plot with

```
> title("Birth weight vs gestational weeks in 500 singleton births")
```

Using indexing for plot elements

One of the most powerful features of R is the possibility to index vectors, not only to get subsets of them, but also to repeat their elements in complex sequences.

Putting separate colours on males and female as above would become very clumsy if we had a 5-level factor instead just two sexes.

Instead of specifying one colour for all points, we may specify a vector of colours of the same length as the gestwks and bweight vectors. This is rather tedious to do directly, but R allows us to specify an expression anywhere, so we can use the fact that sex takes the values 1 and 2, as follows:

First create a colour vector with two colours, and take a look at sex:

```
> c("blue","red")
> births$sex
```

Now see what happens if you index the colour vector by sex:

```
> c("blue","red")[sex]
```

For every occurrence of a 1 in sex you get "blue", and for every occurrence of 2 you get "red", so the result is a long vector of "blue"s and "red"s corresponding to the males and females. This can now be used in the plot:

```
> plot( gestwks, bweight, pch=16, col=c("blue","red")[sex] )
```

The same trick can be used if we want to have a separate symbol for mothers under 30 and over 35, say. We first generate the indexing variable as a factor

```
> magr <- cut( matage, c(0,30,35,100) )
> table( magr )
```

magr is now a factor with 3 levels, and indexing with the variable is the same as indexing with the numerical representation of the factor, 1,2,3; so we ask for symbols 15,16,17 according to the age class of the mother. Moreover, in the specification of the legend we can just use the generated levels as text:

```
> plot( gestwks, bweight, pch=(15:17)[magr], col=c("blue","red")[sex] )
> legend("topleft", pch=15:17, legend=levels(magr), col=1, bty="n")
> text( 28, 4200+0:1*200, c("Boys","Girls"), col=c("blue","red"), adj=0 )
```

Note that we generated the legend for the colours by simply using text to write 'Boys' and 'Girls' in blue and red, respectively.

R will accept any kind of complexity in the indexing as long as the result is a valid index, including a factor.

Interacting with a plot

The `locator()` function allows you to interact with the plot using the mouse. Typing `locator(1)` shifts you to the graphics window and waits for one click of the left mouse button. When you click, it will return the corresponding coordinates.

You can use `locator()` inside other graphics functions to position graphical elements exactly where you want them. Recreate the birth-weight plot,

```
> plot( gestwks, bweight, pch=(15:17)[magr], col=c("blue","red")[sex] )
```

and then add the legend where you wish it to appear by typing:

```
> legend( locator(1), pch=15:17, legend=levels(magr), col=1, bty="n")
> text( locator(2), c("Boys","Girls"), col=c("blue","red"), adj=0 )
```

When `locator` is invoked, the cursor will move to the graphics screen; the first call to `locator` will require one mouse click and the legend will appear at the point. The second call, `locator(2)`, will require two clicks and the two pieces of text will appear where you clicked.

The `identify` function allows you to find out which records in the data correspond to points on the graph. Try

```
> identify( gestwks, bweight )
```

When you click the left mouse button, a label will appear on the graph identifying the row number of the nearest point in the data frame `births`. If there is no point nearby, R will print a warning message on the console instead. To end the interaction with the graphics window, right-click the mouse: the `identify` function returns a vector of identified points—that is the number in the dataset of the points.

Exercises

1. Use `identify()` to find which records correspond to the smallest and largest number of gestational weeks.
2. View all the variables corresponding to these records with

```
births[identify(gestwks, bweight), ]
```

Saving graphs for use in other documents

Once you have a graph in the graphics window in RStudioyou can click on `Export` and choose the format you want your graph in. The `pdf` (Acrobat reader) has a button of its own, `.pdf` normally the most economical, and Acrobat reader has good options for viewing in more detail on the screen.

The `win.metafile` format will give you an enhanced metafile `.emf`, which can be imported into a Word document. Metafiles can be re-sized and edited inside Word; they are in a vector graphics format as are `.pdf` and `.eps`, which means they do not get woolly when enlarged, as do bitmap formats `tiff`, `bmp`, `jpg`, and `png`.

If you want precise control over the size of your plot-file you can start a graphics device *before* doing the plot. Instead of appearing on the screen, the plot will be written directly to a file. After the plot has been completed you will need to close the device again in order to be able to access the file. Try

```
> pdf(file="plot1.pdf", height=3, width=4)
> plot(gestwks, bweight)
> dev.off()
```

This will give you a pdf file `plot1.pdf` with a graph which is 3 inches tall and 4 inches wide. Similarly

```
> win.metafile(file="plot1.emf", height=3, width=4)
> plot(gestwks, bweight)
> dev.off()
```

will give you a emf file `plot1.emf` with a graph which is 3 inches tall and 4 inches wide. This is a vector graphics file that can be inserted in a Word document, and which can be modified in Word.

The `win.metafile` is only available on Windows systems; for other systems, use the device `emf` from the `devEMF` package.

Same graph on multiple devices

If you want the same graph in different file types (or in slightly different aspect ratios), a simple way is to exploit the function facility in R and put the entire plot code into a function with no arguments, and then call the function when different devices are open as in the following example:

```
> myplfn <- function() # Define the function that does the plot
+ {
+ plot( gestwks, bweight, pch=(15:17)[magr], col=c("blue","red")[sex] )
+ legend("topleft", pch=15:17, legend=levels(magr), col=1, bty="n")
+ text( 28, 4200+0:1*200, c("Boys","Girls"), col=c("blue","red"), adj=0 )
+ }
> #
> # on the screen
> myplfn()
> #
> # pdf graph
> pdf( "plot1.pdf", height=8, width=10 )
> myplfn()
> dev.off()
> #
> # windows meta file
> win.metafile( "plot1.eps", height=8, width=10 )
> myplfn()
> dev.off()
```

This has the advantage that if you want to change the plot a little, you only edit the code in one place and all plots will be revised accordingly.

The `par()` command

It is possible to manipulate almost any element in a graph, by using the graphics options. These are collected in the function `par`. For example, if you want axis labels always to be horizontal, use the command `par(las=1)`. This will be in effect until a new graphics device is opened. No one promised you that things should be intuitively clear.

It is a good idea to take a print of the help page for `par` (having set the font size to 'smallest' because it is long) and carry it with you at any time to read in buses, cinema queues, during boring lectures, etc., and perhaps even put under your pillow at night. Do not despair; few R-users can understand what all the options are for.

par can also be used to ask about the current plot; for example par("usr"), will give you the exact extent of the axes in the current plot. With logarithmic axes it's not immediately obvious what you get; you need to read the help page for par.

If you want more plots on a single page you can use the command

```
> par( mfrow=c(2,3) )
```

This will give you a layout of 2 rows by 3 columns for the next 6 graphs you produce. The plots will appear by row, i.e. in the top row first. If you want the plots to appear column-wise, use par(mfcol=c(2,3)) (you still get 2 rows by 3 columns). To restore the layout to a single plot per page use

```
> par( mfrow=c(1,1) )
```

A more versatile machinery for putting multiple graphs on a page in almost arbitrary (rectangular, though) layouts is the function layout—not treated further in this book, but used on p. 140.

1.5 Frequency data

Data from large studies are often summarized in the form of frequency data, which record the frequency of all possible combinations of values of the variables in the study. Such data are sometimes presented in the form of a *contingency* table, sometimes as a data frame in which one variable is the frequency. As an example, consider the UCBAdmissions data, which is one of the standard R datasets, and refers to the outcome of applications to 6 departments at University of California at Berkeley, by gender. The command

```
> str(UCBAdmissions)
 'table' num [1:2, 1:2, 1:6] 512 313 89 19 353 207 17 8 120 205 ...
 - attr(*, "dimnames")=List of 3
  ..$ Admit : chr [1:2] "Admitted" "Rejected"
  ..$ Gender: chr [1:2] "Male" "Female"
  ..$ Dept  : chr [1:6] "A" "B" "C" "D" ...
```

shows that the data are in the form of a $2 \times 2 \times 6$ contingency table for the three variables Admit (Admitted/Rejected), Gender (Male/Female), and Dept (A/B/C/D/E/F).

For convenience in plotting we abbreviate the outcome text:

```
> dimnames(UCBAdmissions)[[1]] <- c("Adm","Rej")
```

CODE EXPLAINED: The dimnames(UCBAdmissions) is a list with three elements, namely the dimension vectors of lengths 2, 2, and 6. If we subset this using [1] we will get a *list* of length 1, which contains the vector ("Admitted","Rejected"). But if we use [[1]], we get the vector itself, which is what we want to replace with a simpler version, namely ("Adm","Rej").

The best way to get an overview of multi-way structures is by using ftable (flat table):

```
> ftable( UCBAdmissions )
              Dept   A   B   C   D   E   F
Admit Gender
Adm   Male          512 353 120 138  53  22
```

```
      Female        89  17 202 131  94  24
Rej   Male         313 207 205 279 138 351
      Female        19   8 391 244 299 317
```

Thus, in department A, 512 males were admitted while 313 were rejected, and so on.

The question of interest is whether there is any bias against admitting female applicants. The following coerces the contingency table to a data frame, and `head` shows the first 6 lines:

```
> ucb <- as.data.frame( UCBAdmissions )
> head(ucb)
  Admit Gender Dept Freq
1   Adm   Male    A  512
2   Rej   Male    A  313
3   Adm Female    A   89
4   Rej Female    A   19
5   Adm   Male    B  353
6   Rej   Male    B  207
```

The relationship between the contingency table and the data frame is that each entry in the contingency table becomes a record in the data frame, with a variable `Freq` holding the entry and the classifications as variables.

The function `effx` that does simple overview analyses will also allow a logical variable as response. We could generate a numerical variable by

```
> rej <- (ucb$Admit=="Rej")*1
```

but this is superfluous, and makes it more difficult to read the code; it is much clearer when the actual condition is listed in the code and the output.

Note that we need to enter the variable `Freq` as the `weight` because each record in the data frame represents `Freq` persons:

```
> effx( response = Admit=="Rej",
+          type = "binary",
+      exposure = Gender,
+        weight = Freq,
+          data = ucb )
-----------------------------------------------------------------
response    :  Admit == "Rej"
type        :  binary
exposure    :  Gender

Gender is a factor with levels: Male / Female
baseline is  Male
effects are measured as odds ratios
-----------------------------------------------------------------

effect of Gender on Admit == "Rej"
number of observations  24

Effect   2.5%  97.5%
  1.84   1.62   2.09

Test for no effects of exposure on 1 df: p-value= <2e-16
```

> CODE EXPLAINED: The first argument to `effx` is the response variable (in this case a logical telling whether a person is denied admission); the second is an indication of what type the response is, in this case binary (TRUE vs FALSE). The third argument is `exposure`, indicating the primary variable of interest, Gender. The `weight` gives the name of the variable that holds the counts, and the final argument `data` indicates in which data frame variables are to be interpreted.

Thus, at first glance it seems that women are some 80% more likely to be rejected, but if we take department (Dept) into account by adding `control=Dept`, it does not seem to be so:

```
> effx( response = Admit=="Rej",
+            type = "binary",
+        exposure = Gender,
+         control = Dept,
+          weight = Freq,
+            data = ucb )
-----------------------------------------------------------------------
response       :  Admit == "Rej"
type           :  binary
exposure       :  Gender
control vars   :  Dept

Gender is a factor with levels: Male / Female
baseline is  Male
effects are measured as odds ratios
-----------------------------------------------------------------------

effect of Gender on Admit == "Rej"
controlled for Dept

number of observations   24

Effect    2.5%   97.5%
 0.905   0.772   1.060

Test for no effects of exposure on 1 df: p-value= 0.216
```

...in fact it looks as women are 10% *less* likely to be rejected—though not 'significantly' so; see p. 53 for a discussion of significance.

What `effx` does here is to fit a statistical model for the admission odds that allows each department its own admission odds, but assuming that the admission odds ratio between women and men within each department is the same across departments. And it is this common odds ratio that is reported. What we see here is a classical example of confounding—department is associated with *both* sex and admission probability, so ignoring department in the analysis will give a distorted picture of the effect of sex per se on admission rates.

If we further look into rejection fractions for women versus men in different departments, replacing `control=Dept` with `strata=Dept`, it seems as if the only department where there is a substantial sex difference is in department A, where women are less likely to be rejected:

```
> effx( response = Admit=="Rej",
+           type = "binary",
+       exposure = Gender,
+         strata = Dept,
+         weight = Freq,
+           data = ucb )
------------------------------------------------------------------
response       :  Admit == "Rej"
type           :  binary
exposure       :  Gender
stratified by  :  Dept

Gender is a factor with levels: Male / Female
baseline is  Male
Dept is a factor with levels: A/B/C/D/E/F
effects are measured as odds ratios
------------------------------------------------------------------

effect of Gender on Admit == "Rej"
stratified by Dept

number of observations   24

                              Effect  2.5% 97.5%
strata A level Female vs Male  0.349 0.209 0.584
strata B level Female vs Male  0.803 0.340 1.890
strata C level Female vs Male  1.130 0.855 1.500
strata D level Female vs Male  0.921 0.686 1.240
strata E level Female vs Male  1.220 0.825 1.810
strata F level Female vs Male  0.828 0.455 1.510

Test for effect modification on 5 df: p-value= 0.00114
```

> CODE EXPLAINED: The first argument to effx is the response variable (in this case a logical telling whether a person is denied admission); the second is an indication of what type the response is, in this case binary (TRUE vs FALSE). The named arguments are exposure, indicating the primary variable of interest; control, indicating a potential confounding variable; and strata, indicating a potential effect modifier. So the two latter uses of effx explore the use of Dept as either confounder or effect modifier. The weight gives the name of the variable that holds the counts.

The final analysis shows that there are differences between departments in the W/M odds ratio of being rejected, although the only one where there is a significantly different rejection rate between men and women is in department A, where women are much *less* likely to be rejected.

From the stratified analysis we see that the departments where women are more likely to be rejected are the departments with the highest proportion of women among applicants.

1.5.1 Graphical overview

We can give a complete graphical overview of the rejection rates between men and women across departments by the function mosaicplot. This function basically draws

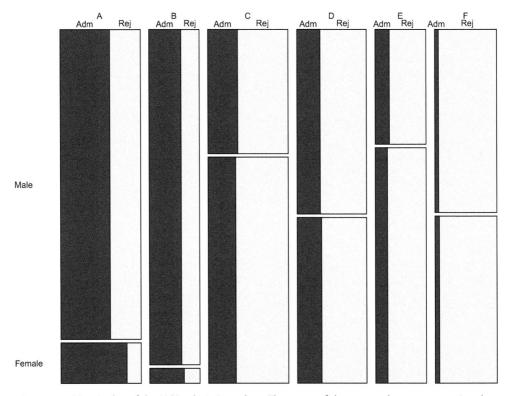

Figure 1.1 Mosaicplot of the UCB admissions data. The areas of the rectangles are proportional to the entries in the table UCBAdmissions.

rectangles with an area proportional to each of the entries in UCBAdmissions, in a clever arrangement (Figure 1.1). It requires a bit of experimentation to get what you want, but the following may be a good approximation to a sensible overview:

```
> par( mar=c(.1,1,1,.1) )
> mosaicplot( UCBAdmissions, sort=3:1, col=TRUE,
+             main="", ylab = "", xlab = "", off=c(0,1,10) )
```

CODE EXPLAINED: The mar argument to par sets the margins of white space around the plot (measured in lines). The 4 numbers refer to bottom, left, top, and right in that order.

The first argument to mosaicplot is a multidimensional (in this case 3-dimensional) table; the sort argument determines in what order the dimension of the table will be considered; col request that the levels of the *last* dimension be coloured in gray-tones. The next three arguments just turns off superfluous annotation, and the off argument determines the amount of space between the rectangles in the plot.

1.5.2 *Ad hoc analyses of admissions*

We can make an ad hoc analysis excluding department A to get an indication of whether the other departments differ w.r.t. admission odds ratio between men and women:

```
> effx( response = Admit=="Rej",
+            type = "binary",
+        exposure = Gender,
+          strata = Dept,
+          weight = Freq,
+            data = transform( subset(ucb, Dept!="A"),
+                              Dept = factor( Dept ) ) )
------------------------------------------------------------------
response       :  Admit == "Rej"
type           :  binary
exposure       :  Gender
stratified by  :  Dept

Gender is a factor with levels: Male / Female
baseline is  Male
Dept is a factor with levels: B/C/D/E/F
effects are measured as odds ratios
------------------------------------------------------------------

effect of Gender on Admit == "Rej"
stratified by Dept

number of observations  20

                                    Effect  2.5% 97.5%
strata B level Female vs Male  0.803 0.340  1.89
strata C level Female vs Male  1.130 0.855  1.50
strata D level Female vs Male  0.921 0.686  1.24
strata E level Female vs Male  1.220 0.825  1.81
strata F level Female vs Male  0.828 0.455  1.51

Test for effect modification on 4 df: p-value= 0.635
```

CODE EXPLAINED: It is not enough to just restrict to the departments not being A, because the variable Dept will still be a factor with A as one of the levels. Therefore we must redefine Dept to a factor with only the actually occurring levels in the subset.

We see that there is no indication of differential rejection rates between departments B–F. However, this p-value is highly biased, because it is based on data where we deliberately excluded a department on the grounds that it was an outlier in a specific direction.

Exercises

1. Use the indexing facility ([,,]) to re-order the sequence of UCB departments by fraction of women applying, thereby creating a mosaicplot with departments ordered by the fraction of women.

1.6 Tables and arrays for results

This section assumes that you are familiar with regression models as described in Chapter 4.2; you can skip this section with no loss of understanding of the subsequent sections.

In the previous section we encountered UCBAdmissions, which was a 3-dimensional table. In R it is possible to define an empty array which is a multidimensional structure similar to a table, but where elements do not have to be numbers, but can be anything.

One use of arrays is to organize results of several parallel analyses. Consider the births data frame, and suppose we wanted to see how bweight and gestwks depend on matage for boys and girls. So for each combination of sex and response variable variable (bweight, getwks) we want to collect the estimate and the confidence intervals of the regression coefficient as well as the p-value. So we set up an array of missing values, classified by the response variables, sex, and with slots for the results:

```
> mA <- NArray( list(resp = c("bweight","gestwks"),
+                    sex = c("M","F"),
+                    res = c("est","lo","hi","P")) )
> str( mA )
 logi [1:2, 1:2, 1:4] NA NA NA NA NA NA ...
 - attr(*, "dimnames")=List of 3
  ..$ resp: chr [1:2] "bweight" "gestwks"
  ..$ sex : chr [1:2] "M" "F"
  ..$ res : chr [1:4] "est" "lo" "hi" "P"
```

We can then use a nested loop to fill the estimates in:

```
> births$sex <- factor( births$sex, labels=c("M","F") )
> for( sx in c("M","F") )
+    {
+ for( rv in c("bweight","gestwks") )
+    {
+    mod <- lm( births[births$sex==sx,rv] ~ births[births$sex==sx,
+    "matage"] ) mA[rv,sx,] <- ci.lin(mod,subset="sex")[,c("Estimate",
+    "2.5%","97.5%","P")]
+    }
+    }
```

CODE EXPLAINED: In order to refer to sex by name we redefine it as a factor with levels as the 2nd dimension in mA. The two nested for loops will cover all 4 combinations of the loop variables sx (sex) and rv (response variable). Inside the loop (between { and }) we fit a model to the subset where sex is equal to the loop variable sx, using the variable rv as response, and matage as explanatory variable. We then use ci.lin to extract the estimate, confidence interval, and p-value. This is a vector of 4 numbers, so we can assign it to mA[rv,sx,], which is also a numerical vector of length 4—if a dimension in an array is referred to by a single value, the corresponding dimension is deleted from the result.

Actually, it is possible to omit the outer set of braces—the two for loops would be nested the same way.

```
> round( ftable(mA), 3 )
> round( ftable(mA,row.vars=2:1), 3 )
> round( ftable(mA,col.vars=1:2), 3 )
```

CODE EXPLAINED: Finally we can print the resulting array mA whichever way we want using the arguments col.vars and row.vars. This flexible printing with ftable is one of the major advantages of collecting analysis results in arrays.

1.7 Dates in R

Epidemiological studies often contain date variables which take values such as 2/11/1962. We shall use the `diet` data to illustrate how to deal with variables whose values are dates.

The important variables in the dataset are `chd`, which takes the value 1 if the subject develops coronary heart disease during the study and 0 if the observation is censored, and the three date variables, which are date of birth (`dob`), date of entry (`doe`), and date of exit (`dox`). The command

```
> data( diet )
> str( diet )
```

shows that these three variables are `Date` variables; if you try

```
> head( diet )
```

you will see these variables printed as 'real' dates. The variables are internally stored as number of days since 1/1/1970.

To convert a character string (or a character variable or factor) to date format try

```
>             as.Date( "14/07/1952", format="%d/%m/%Y" )
> as.numeric( as.Date( "14/07/1952", format="%d/%m/%Y" ) )
```

The first statement shows the date form and the latter the number of days since 1/1/1970, which is a negative number for dates prior to 1/1/1970.

The format parts, '%d' etc., identify elements of the dates, whereas the '/'s are just the separator characters that are in the character string. There is a large number of possibilities for formats; see `?strftime`.

Reading dates from an external file is done by reading the fields as character variables and then transforming them to date variables by the function `as.Date`, using the the relevant format. It will also work if your date variables accidentally ended as factors.

If you want to enter a fixed date, for example if you want to terminate follow-up at 1 April 1995 you could say

```
> newx <- pmin( diet$dox, as.Date( "1995-4-1", format="%F" ) )
```

The format `%F` is shorthand for the ISO-standard date representation `%Y-%m-%d`, which is the default, so it can be omitted altogether:

```
> newx <- pmin( diet$dox, as.Date("1975-4-1") )
```

You will get NAs if your dates are not correct:

```
> as.Date(c("1997-02-28", "1997-02-29", "1997-13-22"))
```

You can have other separators than '-', even quite silly ones:

```
> as.Date( "1995$4$1", format="%Y$%m$%d" )
> as.Date( "1995sep4DIV1", format="%Ysep%mDIV%d" )
```

You can print dates in the format you like by using the function `format` (really `format.Date`); try for example

```
>   bdat <- as.Date( "1952-7-14", format="%F" )
>   format( bdat, format="%A %d %B %Y" )
```

In practical epidemiological analyses it is more convenient to use time measured in years than in days, so the Epi package has a function cal.yr that converts dates to numeric years

```
> ( dd <- as.Date(c('1970-1-1',
+                   '1971-1-1',
+                   '1972-1-1',
+                   '1973-1-1',
+                   '1974-1-1',
+                   '1975-1-1')) )
[1] "1970-01-01" "1971-01-01" "1972-01-01" "1973-01-01" "1974-01-01"
[6] "1975-01-01"
> cal.yr(dd)
[1] 1970.000 1970.999 1971.999 1973.001 1974.000 1974.999
attr(,"class")
[1] "cal.yr"  "numeric"
```

Because of the leap years it is only every 4th year 1 January precisely fits with an integer. Formally, the cal.yr converts dates (measured in units of days) to units of 365.25 days, and we just choose to call this unit 'year'. The conventional use of 'year' is formally inaccurate, because a year sometimes is 365 and sometimes 366 days.

You can also see that the differences between the dates are not the same, neither measured in days or 'years' of course:

```
> diff( dd )
> diff( cal.yr(dd) )
```

On the other hand if you take dates that have a given distance in days you get consistency:

```
> ( xx <- as.Date("1970-1-17")+0:5*300 )
[1] "1970-01-17" "1970-11-13" "1971-09-09" "1972-07-05" "1973-05-01"
[6] "1974-02-25"
> diff( cal.yr(xx) )
[1] 0.8213552 0.8213552 0.8213552 0.8213552 0.8213552
attr(,"class")
[1] "cal.yr"  "numeric"
```

In the package lubridate there is a function decimal_date that appears to do the same, but is slightly inconsistent for epidemiological purposes:

```
> library( lubridate )
>       decimal_date(xx)
[1] 1970.044 1970.866 1971.688 1972.508 1973.329 1974.151
> diff( decimal_date(xx) )
[1] 0.8219178 0.8219178 0.8205255 0.8205704 0.8219178
```

Even if the 6 dates in xx are equidistant, using decimal_date renders them non-equidistant, so decimal_date provides a non-linear transformation of dates. The non-linearity is small, but it is indeed an odd measurement unit for time that is 365 days in non-leap years and 366 days in leap years.

A similar odd behaviour is obtained from the function get.yrs in the popEpi package, which does calculations in two different ways, where actual corresponds to the behaviour of decimal_date:

```
> library(popEpi)
> diff( get.yrs( xx, year.length="actual" ) )
[1] 0.8219178 0.8219178 0.8205255 0.8205704 0.8219178
> diff( get.yrs( xx, year.length="approx" ) )
[1] 0.8213728 0.8220359 0.8220359 0.8192980 0.8220359
```

So neither `decimal_date` nor `get.yrs` should be used in practical epidemiology. More out of principle than because of the added inaccuracy, which is quite small. Adding unnecessary error to your data, however small, is generally discouraged.

In addition to common sanity, `cal.yr` has the facility that with a data frame as argument it will find all `Date` variables in the data frame and convert them to `cal.yr` format, and return the data frame with the converted variables; try

```
> data(diet)
> diet[1:4,1:4]
     id        doe        dox        dob
1 102 1976-01-17 1986-12-02 1939-03-02
2  59 1973-07-16 1982-07-05 1912-07-05
3 126 1970-03-17 1984-03-20 1919-12-24
4  16 1969-05-16 1969-12-31 1906-09-17
> food <- cal.yr(diet)
> food[1:4,1:4]
     id      doe      dox      dob
1 102 1976.042 1986.917 1939.164
2  59 1973.537 1982.507 1912.508
3 126 1970.205 1984.215 1919.977
4  16 1969.370 1969.997 1906.709
> str( food[1:4] )
'data.frame':    337 obs. of  4 variables:
 $ id : num   102 59 126 16 247 272 268 206 182 2 ...
 $ doe: 'cal.yr' num   1976 1974 1970 1969 1968 ...
 $ dox: 'cal.yr' num   1987 1983 1984 1970 1979 ...
 $ dob: 'cal.yr' num   1939 1913 1920 1907 1919 ...
```

Exercises

1. Generate a new variable `y` which is the elapsed time in years between the date of entry and the date of exit.
2. Enter your own birthday as a date. Print it using `format.Date()` with the format `"%A %d %B %Y"`. Did you learn anything new?
3. Print your birthday in `cal.yr` format.
4. Enter the birthday of your husband/wife/... as a date too. When will you be (or were you) 100 years old together? (Hint: `mean()` works on vectors of dates as well.)

1.8 Numerical accuracy

Computers are not mathematically accurate; there is some inaccuracy in the representation of numbers. Although the expression below should give 1, and seems to do that, A is not equal to 1 according to R. Note that we put a set of brackets around the assignment to A which is a handy way of printing the value of the assignment:

```
> b <- 8349174
> a <- 8745134
> ( A <- (a/b)*(b/a) )
[1] 1
> A == 1
[1] FALSE
```

So even if quantity prints as 1, it is not necessarily equal to 1. The general advice for quantitative variables is that you should not ask whether their value is equal to some fixed quantity (such as 0 or 1), but whether the absolute difference from it is smaller than some suitably tiny number:

```
> abs( A-1 ) < 1e-12
[1] TRUE
```

A more handy way of doing this is via the function `near` in the `dplyr` package:

```
> library( dplyr )
> near( A, 1 )
[1] TRUE
```

1.8.1 *Accuracy of matching variables*

The (lack of) numerical inaccuracy is of importance when merging datasets on a common identification variable, constructed as a 15- or 20-digit number, say. This should not be used for matching; instead, a character version of the identification variable should be used; this will always produce an exact match. You should convert to a character identification variable when you read data; trying after the fact may give undesired results:

```
> cat("747546743584815682   83.6
+       747546743584815765 102.7\n", file = "xx.txt")
> #
> df <- read.table( "xx.txt", colClasses=c('character','numeric') )
> df[1,1] == df[2,1]
[1] FALSE
> df
                   V1    V2
1 747546743584815682  83.6
2 747546743584815765 102.7
> #
> df <- read.table( "xx.txt", colClasses=c('numeric','numeric') )
> df
           V1    V2
1 7.475467e+17  83.6
2 7.475467e+17 102.7
> df[1,1] == df[2,1]
[1] TRUE
> as.character(df[1,1]) == as.character(df[2,1])
[1] TRUE
> as.character(df[,1])
[1] "747546743584815744" "747546743584815744"
```

CODE EXPLAINED: The cat function just prints the first argument to a file, in this case xx.txt; the last \n is merely a newline. The point here is to print two very long numbers that only differ in the last 3 digits. When you read the data using read.table with colClasses (column Classes) to indicate that the first column is character and the second numerical, R can actually distinguish the two long numbers; well, not numbers, they are actually character strings.

But if you pretend they are numerical, R cannot tell the difference between the two numbers—numbers are only represented to a certain precision in a computer.

The last attempt to resurrect the variables as character fails because they are already inaccurately represented as numerical from the reading. But if these large numbers were person ids the results from as.character would look deceptively like a valid id, even if it were nowhere to be found in the original file.

Moral: If you want to have precise representation (for example, when merging files on an id variable), always use a character representation. Numeric variables are those you plan to do arithmetic operations on—quantitative variables.

A devoted purist would only ever match on character variables or factors.

1.9 tidyverse and data.table

The people at RStudio have developed a package dplyr with an expanded data frame concept (called a tibble) which also allows the use of data.table, the latter an independent extension of data frames. dplyr is part of the collection of interconnected packages called tidyverse (for some reason often called 'an ecosystem') that also comprise the ggplot2 package and packages such as plyr, dbplyr, tidyr, primarily aimed at data management and what is termed data science. tidyverse presents a syntax for data manipulation tasks, different from the standard R, but fully integrated.

These packages contain a number of useful functions, extending the operations available in the indexing of data frames, as well as a number of more advanced data manipulation and summarizing functions.

A description can be found at https://r4ds.had.co.nz/index.html, which is basically an online version of the book *R for Data Science* from the publisher O'Reilly. Other very good introductions to these tools exist in the packages themselves in the form of vignettes—articles explaining the concepts, in either html or pdf format. You can access these by

```
> library( dplyr )
> browseVignettes(package = "dplyr")
> library( data.table )
> browseVignettes(package = "data.table")
```

This is, however, a book on epidemiology with R, not about data manipulation, so we shall not venture into these topics further.

CHAPTER 2

Measures of disease occurrence

This chapter gives a brief introduction to some of the most common measures of disease occurrence used in epidemiology, both the empirical and theoretical versions of the measures.

More elaborate exposition of the statistics of proportions and rates are given in Chapters 3 and 5, respectively.

2.1 Prevalence

The prevalence of a disease in a population is the fraction of the population that has the disease at a given date. Therefore, the prevalence always refers to a specific point in time, usually a date like 1 January 2010.

The total number of persons in Denmark alive with colon cancer as of 1 January 2010 was 16,281, and the number of persons in Denmark on 1 January 2010 was 5,534,738, so the prevalence of colon cancer is

```
> 16281/5534738
[1] 0.002941603
```

that is, 0.29%.

This is the *empirical prevalence* of colon cancer patients in the Danish population—the actual fraction of the population with a diagnosis of colorectal cancer on 1 January 2010.

The *theoretical prevalence* is the probability that a randomly chosen person from the population has colorectal cancer. This is an unknown quantity, but a reasonable estimate of it would be the the empirical prevalence. That is, however, just an *estimate* from a statistical model that asserts that colon cancer is randomly distributed among all Danes with probability p, where

$$p = \mathrm{P}\{\text{randomly chosen person has colon cancer}\}$$

There is an uncertainty associated with the *estimate*, which we can quantify in a *confidence interval*. This is an interval that captures the true prevalence, p, with some prespecified probability; normally 95% is used.

An elaborate explanation of the statistical models underlying this type of calculation for prevalence is given in Chapter 3.

The *data* used to estimate p are X=number of persons with colorectal cancer, and N=number of persons in the population. In order to assess p we can fit a binomial model (this is explained in detail in Chapter 3):

Epidemiology with R. Bendix Carstensen, Oxford University Press (2021). © Bendix Carstensen.
DOI: 10.1093/oso/9780198841326.003.0003

```
> library( Epi )
> X <- 16281
> N <- 5554738
> mp <- glm( cbind( X, N-X ) ~ 1, family=binomial )
> round( ci.pred( mp ) * 100, 4 )
  Estimate   2.5%  97.5%
1   0.2942 0.2897 0.2987
```

> CODE EXPLAINED: glm fits a generalized linear model, in this case a model for a binomial outcome (family=binomial). The observed outcome must be specified as the number of successes (X, number of diseased) and the number of failures (N-X, number of non-diseased; note *not* the total number). The prevalence as a function of explanatory variables is described by a *model*, here specified by ~1, which means that the prevalence is constant across all observational units (not surprisingly so, since we only have one data point). The ci.pred produces a prediction of the theoretical prevalence from the model with a 95% confidence interval.

2.2 Mortality rate

Mortality is typically reported as a number of people that have died in a population of a certain size: '2,648 persons died out of 150,000 persons'. This is a mortality of 17.6 per 1,000 persons, apparently:

```
> 2648 / 150000
[1] 0.01765333
```

Looking a bit closer at this, it is bit illogical—the number of deaths (2,648) must be recorded over some period of time, in this case presumably a year. The number of persons, on the other hand, refer to the population size at some specific date, presumably 1st January or July some year. So the two components, number of deaths and population size, refer to a *period* and a specific *time point*, respectively.

The number of persons at risk of dying will not vary a lot over a year, so as a first approximation we might assume that the population was constant in the period. Thus, the 150,000 above refers to the *average* population over the period.

But if the 2,648 deaths were accumulated over a period of two years, the mortality would then be half of what we just computed, because the 150,000 people had each had two years to encounter death. This leads to the concept of *person-years*—also called risk time, time at risk, exposed time, or even just exposure (the latter mostly used in demography). The person-years is the population size multiplied by the length of the observation interval. So since the population size is 150,000 and the observation period is 2 years, the number of person-years is 300,000, and the mortality rate is $2,648/300,000 = 8.83$ deaths per 1,000 person-years:

```
> 2648/300
[1] 8.826667
```

Note that the rate is a *scaled* quantity—it has a *unit* of measurement, in this example 'per 1000 PY'. We might equally well have given the mortality rate as 88.3 per 10,000 person-years.

This quantity is what we call the *empirical* mortality rate. The *theoretical* counterpart is the probability of dying in a small interval, *relative* to the length of the interval. This is usually denoted by the Greek letter lambda, λ:

$$\lambda = P\{\text{death in } (t, t + dt) \mid \text{alive at } t\} / dt$$

When we say 'small' interval, we are approcaching the formal definition as the limit of the quantity as dt tends to 0; dt is just mathematical jargon for a small piece of the t-scale.

The vertical bar denotes *conditional* probability (pronounced 'given'). Note that the theoretical rate is also a scaled quantity; it is measured in units of time^{-1}—deaths per person-time—because the denominator dt is measured in time units.

As in the case of prevalence, there is an uncertainty associated with the estimate of the theoretical mortality rate, which we can quantify in a *confidence interval*.

The *data* used to estimate λ are D=number of deaths, and Y=amount of follow-up time. In order to assess this we can fit a Poisson model—the likelihood for survival data has the same form as the likelihood for Poisson data (see Chapter 5 for a detailed explanation of this):

```
> library( Epi )
> D <- 2648
> Y <- 300000
> mm <- glm( D ~ 1, offset=log(Y), family=poisson )
> round( ci.pred( mm, newdata=data.frame(Y=1000) ), 3 )
  Estimate  2.5% 97.5%
1    8.827 8.497 9.169
```

CODE EXPLAINED: glm fits a generalized linear model, in this case a model for a Poisson outcome (family=poisson). The observed outcome is the number of deaths (D), and the amount of follow-up time (Y), the latter specified in the offset argument. The mortality rate is described through a *model* for the *number* of events. The model is here specified by ~1, which means that the mortality rate is constant over all observed units— specifically, that the number of deaths is proportional to the number of person-years as supplied in the offset argument. The ci.pred predicts the expected number of deaths for a specified value of Y, in this case, 1,000. Since the Y was entered in the model in units of person-years, the prediction will be for 1,000 person-years when we set Y equal to 1,000 when predicting. The result is therefore an estimate of the mortality rate *per 1,000 person-years*. Mortality rates in the range 8.5–9.2 per 1,000 person-years are therefore seen as consistent with an observation of 2,648 deaths in 300,000 person-years.

In the Epi package you will find the so-called 'family' poisreg specifically designed for analysis of rates. It fits the Poisson model (or rather maximizes the Poisson likelihood), but uses a more intuitive notation (similar to the binomial), namely events and person-years as a two-column matrix:

```
> mr <- glm( cbind(D,Y/1000) ~ 1, family=poisreg )
> round( ci.pred( mr, newdata=data.frame(x=NA) ), 3 )
  Estimate  2.5% 97.5%
1    8.827 8.497 9.169
> round( ci.pred( mr ), 3 )
  Estimate  2.5% 97.5%
1    8.827 8.497 9.169
```

> CODE EXPLAINED: The family `poisreg` has the events (D) and risk time (Y) as response variables, so the person-years are not needed in the prediction frame. This means that the scaling of rates is done when specifying the response—basically we must decide whether we are modelling rates per 1 PY or (as here) rates per 1,000 PY. Since there are no covariates in the model, we only use the `newdata` argument to determine the size of the prediction vector; the names and the values of columns in the `newdata` data frame are irrelevant: the only thing used is the number of rows (in this case, 1). The `x=NA` is just to specify a non-empty data frame, but `ci.pred` allows `newdata` to be left unspecified if the model has no covariates.

We shall use the `poisreg` family as the main tool for the analysis of rates in the rest of this book.

2.3 Incidence rate

Incidence rates are defined exactly as mortality rates, where we just count *incident cases*, that is, newly diagnosed cases of a particular disease.

In chronic disease epidemiology, persons are removed from the risk set once they acquire the disease, so the person-years are only counted for those without the disease. For diseases which may recur (such as leg fractures, for example), persons may re-enter the risk population either immediately or after some specified grace period. Definition of a grace period is a subject-matter question.

If the prevalence of a disease is small (e.g. lung cancer), the difference between the non-diseased part of the population and the total population is negligible, so the distinction is of little practical relevance. But if the prevalence is high—for example, diabetes prevalence in elderly persons is typically in the vicinity of 15%—it is essential to use person-years among non-affected persons only. Otherwise, the incidence rates will be underestimated.

2.4 Standardized mortality ratio

The standardized mortality ratio (SMR) is a measure of the mortality in a group of persons (for example, a particular occupation such as bus drivers) as compared to the general population. Originally, the term referred to a particular procedure that compared the *observed* number of deaths (*O*) in a study group with the *expected* number of deaths (*E*) in the group to form the SMR = *O/E*. The expected number is computed assuming the population rates, which makes the SMR an estimate of the mortality rate ratio between the study group and the general population.

In contemporary literature SMR is increasingly used as a synonym for the mortality rate ratio even if the calculation is done through a statistical model.

If population incidence rates (of, say, cancer) are available, similar calculations of the expected number of incident cases can be done. In these instances it has become customary to refer to the ratio of observed to expected numbers as SIR, standardized *incidence* ratio, though some still use the term SMR as an abbreviation of standardized *morbidity* ratio.

2.5 Survival

The survival after diagnosis of a disease is defined as the fraction of diagnosed individuals alive at a given time after diagnosis. Direct calculation of this at, say, 2 years requires that the entire group of diagnosed patients has been followed for at least 2 years.

In that case we are just looking at the prevalence of 2-year survivors among the diagnosed persons followed for at least 2 years. So for complete data the empirical and theoretical survival fractions are defined as prevalences, those surviving 2 years and the probability that a randomly chosen patient survives 2 years, respectively.

If not all of the patients are observed for, say, 2 years, techniques for *censored* survival data must be used; see Chapter 8.

Note that survival requires a well-defined *origin* as opposed to a calculation of rates—we are talking about the probability of surviving a given time *after* some specific time-point, often the diagnosis of a disease.

If there is a well-defined origin of the time-scale from which we have observed deaths, there is a one-to-one correspondence between survival and mortality, which also allows mortality to vary by time (since origin). If $S(t)$ is the survival at time t, then the formal relation between survival and rates is

$$S(t) = \exp\left(-\int_0^t \lambda(s)\, ds\right) \quad \Leftrightarrow \quad \lambda(t) = \frac{-d\log\left(S(t)\right)}{dt}$$

Thus if we have (or are willing to arbitrarily define) an origin we can establish a one-to-one relationship between survival and mortality rate. Conversely, we can say that a survival function requires an origin and a rate function.

2.5.1 *Cumulative risk*

The cumulative risk of death is just 1− the survival probability. For a non-fatal condition the cumulative risk is the probability of the event occurring before a given time t, which depends not only on the occurrence rate of the condition in question, but also on the mortality rate for persons without the condition. This is treated in the section on competing risks, section 8.8.

2.5.2 *Competing risks*

Competing risks is the designation of the situation where a person can die from different causes, or where different diseases and death compete for events. Basically it is the situation where more than one type of event can happen; this can be completely described by the type-specific occurrence rates. The cause-specific rates are estimated by relating events of different types to the population risk time. These can be modelled separately, and covariate effects are estimated exactly as in an analysis of rates (see Chapter 8); the only difference is that persons who see an event of a different type than the one in question should be censored at the time of the other event.

It is only in estimating the cumulative risk of a given event type that the rates of other types of events are used. The analysis of a cause-specific rate is only based on the events of the specific type, while events of other types and censorings are all treated as censorings.

2.5.3 *Sojourn time*

This is the term for the time spent in a certain condition or state. For example, we may ask what is the expected time (during the remaining life-span) spent with, respectively without, heart disease for a man aged 50. This can only be formulated precisely in a multistate model with transition rates between different states (including death)—the relevant states here would be 'Alive with heart disease', 'Alive without heart disease' and 'Dead'. Normally sojourn time in death states is not counted, but in priciple it makes sense as lifetime lost—you may recall the remark by Tom Lehrer: 'It's a sobering thought, for example, that when Mozart was my age, he had been dead for two years.'

Sojourn times can be derived from a complete specification of all transition rates between different states and death, but this is again a topic in the realm of multistate modelling which is outside the scope of this book.

CHAPTER 3

Prevalence data—models, likelihood, and binomial regression

Prevalence of a disease condition in a population is merely the proportion of affected people. Here we use prevalence to illustrate core modelling concepts: the model itself, the likelihood, the maximum likelihood estimation principle, and the properties of the results, all of which underlies most modern epidemiological methods.

The dataset pr is available in the Epi package:

```
> library( Epi )
> data( pr )
> str( pr )
'data.frame':   200 obs. of  4 variables:
 $ A  : num  0 0 10 10 11 11 12 12 13 13 ...
 $ sex: Factor w/ 2 levels "M","F": 2 1 2 1 2 1 2 1 2 1 ...
 $ X  : num  1 0 84 83 106 70 104 111 133 120 ...
 $ N  : num  30743 32435 32922 34294 32890 ...
```

It contains the number of diabetes patients (X) and the total number of persons in Denmark (N) as of 1 January 2010, classified by age (A, 0,1,2,...,99) and sex (sex, M,F). We shall use this for illustration of the principle of likelihood estimation and the concept of a statistical model leading to the distinction between *empirical* and *theoretical* prevalences.

3.1 Likelihood

3.1.1 *A single probability*

If we look at 60-year-old men:

```
> subset( pr, sex=="M" & A==60 )
    A sex   X     N
114 60   M 3632 34416
```

we see that prevalence is 3,632 cases out of 34,416 persons, so 3632/34416 = 0.1055323 or some 10.6% (the first number printed is just the record number in the dataset). We can think of the 10.6% as a quantity that governs an experiment where we randomly select a 60-year-old man (out of the 34,416 available at 1 January 2010) and ask whether he has diabetes. The probability of a 'yes' is then 10.6%. This way we have an experiment where

Epidemiology with R. Bendix Carstensen, Oxford University Press (2021). © Bendix Carstensen.
DOI: 10.1093/oso/9780198841326.003.0004

we *know* what to expect; we know that the probability is 10.6%. So in this sense we know the probability machinery that generates our data.

But in most real settings the situation is the other way round; we have the collected data, and we want to know something about the machinery that generated the data.

When we establish the experiment of selecting a random person and determining his diabetes status we would like to know what the likely outcome is. If we *know* that in the entire population (as we do) the probability of 'yes' is 10.6% we know how the experiment will pan out, but suppose we did not know this and could only survey, say, 100 men aged 60. We would then have the problem that we would like to say something about the 'true' prevalence based on a small sample. So let us take a sample of 100 men aged 60 from our population:

```
> set.seed( 1952 )
> rbinom( 1, 100, 0.1055323 )
[1] 16
```

> CODE EXPLAINED: set.seed sets a starting point for the random number generator (which has the effect that the code will generate the same random number(s) each time it is run). rbinom generates one (1, the first argument) random number from the binomial distribution with parameters ($n = 100$, $p = 0.1055323$), that is, the result of 100 draws, each with probability 0.1055323.

So from the 16 diabetes cases seen among the 100 randomly selected men we will try to determine the fraction of *all* 60-year-old men that have diabetes, that is, to say something about the population we got the data from. A good guess is of course 16%—the empirical or observed fraction in our sample.

There is a theoretical basis for this guess; suppose the true (but unknown) fraction is π, then the probability of seeing 16 out of 100 is

$$l(\pi) = P\{16 \text{ out of } 100\} = \binom{100}{16} \pi^{16}(1 - \pi)^{100-16}$$

The probability regarded as a function of the parameter π is called the *likelihood* (of the observed data). The first term is the binomial coefficient, telling how many ways you can choose 16 from a set of 100. For any value of π this probability is a really tiny number, but we will choose the value of π that makes this probability (the likelihood of the data) as large as possible. In other words, choose a prevalence guess among all possible πs that makes our observation the most likely—hence, the term maximum likelihood.

Note that there are 100 terms, 16 terms with a π and 84 with a $(1 - \pi)$, and that these are multiplied. This makes up the probability of observing one particular configuration of the presence and absence of diabetes among 100 persons, but only under the assumption that the 100 persons we look at are *independent*. This would, for example, not be the case if some of the persons were related and there was a substantial familiar component to diabetes.

Finding the value of π for which the probability is maximal is the same as finding the π for which the log of the probability is maximal. We use the log-likelihood because this is a *sum* of terms instead of a product, and so much easier to handle from a mathematical point of view.

So we look at the log of the likelihood, ℓ (where K is the log of the binomial coefficient, which does not depend on π):

$$\ell(\pi) = \log\left(P\{16 \text{ out of } 100\}\right) = 16\log(\pi) + 84\log(1 - \pi) + K$$

It turns out that the value of π that maximizes this function is indeed $\pi = 16/100$—not surprisingly the intuitive choice. If we had observed x out of n we would have found x/n as the value for π that makes the log-likelihood (and hence the probability of the observed data) as large as possible. The convention is to label the maximum likelihood estimate $\hat{\pi}$, so we just derived that for our sample, $\hat{\pi} = 16/100$.

This seems a long detour for a rather trivial result, but the point is that the maximum likelihood principle can be generalized to more complex situations, in particular situations with more than one parameter. For more complex situations it suffices to know that it is possible to compute the probability of seeing the observed data at the maximum likelihood value of the model parameters—normally termed the likelihood of the fitted model.

3.1.2 Simple confidence interval

Another benefit of this general method is that the underlying theory allows us to attach uncertainty to the estimate.[1] A general rule is that if we take minus the inverse of the 2nd derivative of the log-likelihood with respect to π and evaluate it for $\pi = \hat{\pi}$ we get the variance of the estimate. The standard error of the estimate is then the square root of this.

If we do the mathematics of this, it turns out that in the binomial distribution

$$\text{s.e.}(\hat{\pi}) = \sqrt{\pi(1-\pi)/n}$$

and so we can derive a confidence interval for the estimated prevalence as (replacing π with $\hat{\pi}$ as the best guess we have)

$$\hat{\pi} \pm 2\sqrt{\hat{\pi}(1-\hat{\pi})/n}$$

Here we have boldly used the approximation 2 to the 97.5 percentile of the normal distribution—the usual one used is 1.96.

This confidence interval for a probability has the unfortunate drawback that one of the bounds may fall outside the interval $[0, 1]$; this happens if x is very small. Using the data from our example we get

```
> n <- 100
> x <- 16
> p <- x/n
> se <- sqrt(p*(1-p)/100)
> round( c( p, p-2*se, p+2*se ), 4 )
[1] 0.1600 0.0867 0.2333
```

so in this case we get a reasonable confidence interval, incidentally containing the true parameter ($\pi = 10.9\%$) used in the simulation—an event which occurs with (approximately) 95% probability. But if we had seen 3 out of 25, we would get an illogical result:

```
> P <- 3/25
> SE <- sqrt(P*(1-P)/25)
> round( c( P, P-2*SE, P+2*SE ), 4 )
[1]  0.12 -0.01  0.25
```

---

[1] Here we will use the concept of a confidence interval which will be explained in section 3.1.3, p. 51.

We see that the lower bound of the confidence intervals is negative—not very sensible for a probability that necessarily is between 0 and 1. To remedy this, we might instead calculate some function of the prevalence π and the standard error of this; construct a confidence interval for this function of π and then transform back. If we choose the function carefully we can get something that always provides a sane result.

It turns out that a good choice of transformation is the log-*odds*, $\theta = \log(\pi/(1 - \pi)) \Leftrightarrow \pi = 1/(1 + \exp(-\theta))$. This function that converts from probability to log-odds is called *logit*.

Similarly to the conversion between probabilities and odds (p. 8) we can devise functions that convert both ways between probability and log-odds:

```
> logit <- function( p ) log( p / (1-p) )
> tigol <- function( t ) 1 / ( 1 + exp(-t) )
```

(tigol is just the letters of logit reversed).

The log-odds has the property that when π moves from 0 to 1, the log.odds moves from $-\infty$ to $+\infty$. Doing the mathematics[2] for the standard error of θ will give

$$\text{s.e.}(\theta) = \text{s.e.} \left(\log\left(\pi/(1-\pi)\right) \right) = 1/\sqrt{n\pi(1-\pi)} = \sqrt{\frac{1}{x} + \frac{1}{n-x}} \qquad (3.1)$$

where the last equal sign is using $x = n\pi$ as a convenience.

This can be used to form a confidence interval for the log-odds, θ, that can be transformed back to a confidence interval for the probability:

$$\theta \pm 1.96 \times 1/\sqrt{n\pi(1-\pi)}$$

If we use this on our data we get

```
> lo   <- logit( p )
> loS <- 1 / sqrt ( n * p * (1-p) )
> loL <- lo - 1.96 * loS
> loU <- lo + 1.96 * loS
> round( tigol( c(lo,loL,loU) ), 3 )

[1] 0.160 0.100 0.245
```

We see that the log-odds-based interval (10.0;24.5)% is a little closer to 0.5 than the intuitive one we started with—this will always be the case.

But the logit transformation will remedy the problem we saw with 3 out of 25:

```
> n <- 25 ; x <- 3 ; p <- x/n
> lo   <- logit( p )
> loS <- 1 / sqrt ( n * p * (1-p) )
> loL <- lo - 1.96 * loS
> loU <- lo + 1.96 * loS
> round( tigol( c(lo,loL,loU) ), 3 )

[1] 0.120 0.039 0.313
```

So we have derived an estimated prevalence of diabetes for 60-year-old men and an uncertainty of this in the form of a confidence interval. This is based on a statistical *model* where we postulate a random mechanism (binomial distribution) that generated

---

[2] Express the log-likelihood in terms of θ, derive the 2nd derivative w.r.t. θ, and express the result in terms of π.

the data and estimated a parameter (the probability that a randomly selected 60-year-old man has diabetes). This parameter is what we would call the *theoretical* prevalence of diabetes among 60-year-old men. It represents the probability that a randomly chosen 60-year-old man in the population has diabetes.

3.1.3 *Confidence intervals in general*

In the mainstream frequentist school of statistics we are formally using a probability statement about the confidence *interval*. This states that there is a fixed, non-random, but unknown value of the parameter and the randomness connected with the calculation of the confidence interval is such that there is a (say) 95% probability that the interval covers the true value. Many people find this hard to grasp, and some have even learned to reproduce this convoluted statement.

Most people think of a confidence interval for a parameter as a range of credible values for the parameter, where the location and size of the interval is derived from the data base. Like we just did above. This can be formalized in the Bayesian school of statistics where parameters are not taken as true fixed quantities, but rather regarded as random variables. If a parameter is considered a random variable it is sensible to produce probability statements about it, such as 'there is 95% probability that π is in the interval (π_L, π_U)'. Bayesians call it 'credible intervals' instead of 'confidence intervals'.

The Bayesian way is presumably the way most people think of confidence/credible intervals, but they have also learned that it is formally wrong, and do not speak the heretical words. In reality the difference between the two approaches is minimal; with suitable assumptions we can almost always make the Bayesian credible intervals effectively coincide with the frequentist confidence intervals.

3.1.4 *The normal distribution*

The technical side of confidence interval calculation is based on the central limit theorem, which broadly speaking asserts that if a random quantity is derived from many small random sources, it is approximately normally distributed. The normal distribution is also called the Gaussian distribution.[3] This means that if we can get our hands on the standard error (the square root of the variance) of a parameter, a good approximation to a 95% confidence interval is the parameter value ± 2 standard error. The number 2 is a characteristic of the normal distribution; just about 95% of the probability mass in the normal distribution is within ± 2 standard errors from the mean:

```
> pnorm(q=2,mean=0,sd=1) - pnorm(q=-2,mean=0,sd=1)
[1] 0.9544997
> c( qnorm(p=0.025), qnorm(p=0.975) )
[1] -1.959964  1.959964
> c( qnorm(p=0.05) , qnorm(p=0.95) )
[1] -1.644854  1.644854
```

---

[3] After Carl Friederich Gauss, 1777–1855, a German scientist to whom the least-squares method is usually ascribed. Least-squares estimation corresponds to maximum likelihood estimation in the normal distribution. The Gaussian distribution was shown alongside a portrait of Gauss on the 10 Deutsch Mark bank note prior to institution of the Euro in 2000.

> CODE EXPLAINED: pnorm computes the probability that a normally distributed variate is less than q (the first argument to the function). So the first statement computes the probability that a normally distributed variate is between 2 standard errors above (q=2) the mean and 2 standard errors below (q=-2) the mean.
>
> qnorm finds the point q in the normal distribution where the probability of being less than q is p (the first argument to the function), so a 95% confidence interval will rigorously be using $\pm1.96\times$ standard error, and a 90% confidence interval using $\pm1.64\times$ standard error.

The practical calculation of confidence intervals uses the assumption of a normal distribution of the parameter and computes a confidence interval as the estimate plus/minus twice the standard error.

3.1.5 *Simple confidence intervals from models*

The log-odds is also what is estimated by default in binomial models—normally called logistic regression.

We can fit a logistic regression to our simple data to show that we can reproduce the simple results as special cases of a more general model. We use the glm function which fits generalized linear models, of which the logistic regression model is one. The log-odds is the default parameter estimated when we specify the binomial distribution. Note that in R the response in a binomial model must be a two-column matrix, with the first column containing the number of successes and the second the number of failures (*not* the total number of trials), hence the specification cbind(x,n-x):

```
> x <- 16
> n <- 100
> m0 <- glm( cbind(x,n-x) ~ 1, family = binomial(link=logit) )
> round( ci.lin(m0), 4 )
            Estimate StdErr      z P    2.5%    97.5%
(Intercept)  -1.6582 0.2728 -6.0792 0 -2.1929 -1.1236
> c( log(16/84), 1/sqrt(100*0.16*0.84) )
[1] -1.6582281  0.2727724
```

> CODE EXPLAINED: glm fits a binomial model to the data which is 16 events (x) in 100 trials (n), and ci.lin extracts the parameter which is the log-odds. We see that the parameter indeed is the log-odds, and that the hand-computed standard error is the one derived by glm.

We can back transform from the log-odds (logit) scale by using the inverse logit function we just defined (tigol, see p. 50):

```
> round( tigol( ci.lin(m0)[,c(1,5,6)] ), 4 )
Estimate    2.5%    97.5%
  0.1600  0.1004   0.2453
```

> CODE EXPLAINED: Since the results is on the log-odds scale, we need a transformation to get the probability. This is done with the inverse logit-function tigol, defined on p. 50. We see that we get the same as we got by using the explicit formulae.

In the code on p. 52 we used `link=logit` which is actually superfluous, because it is the default for the binomial family to model the log-odds ('logit'). But we could have used the log-link instead:

```
> ml <- glm( cbind(x,n-x) ~ 1, family = binomial(link=log) )
> ci.exp(ml)
                exp(Est.)     2.5%      97.5%
(Intercept)         0.16 0.102114 0.2507002
```

> CODE EXPLAINED: `glm` with `family=binomial(link=log)` fits a binomial model as well; however, the parameter is not the log-*odds*, but the log-*probability*, so `ci.exp` will directly produce the estimated prevalence.

We get the same estimates, but slightly different confidence limits because we are using a normal approximation to the log-probability instead of an approximation to the log-odds as above.

Thus, even the simplest proportions can be estimated using a statistical model, and the confidence intervals comes along at virtually no extra cost. A further reason to do this is to ensure the capability of expanding to more complex settings.

3.1.6 Tests and p-values

Hypothesis testing is widespread in the clinical literature, and unfortunately also in the epidemiological. In the previous example we found (by simulation) 16 diabetes patients among 100 men aged 60. We simulated from a binomial distribution with probability 0.1055, so we know where the data came from. But if we did not know we could ask the question of whether the data (16 out of 100) were reasonably compatible with a true underlying prevalence of 10%? Or more precisely whether the theoretical prevalence can be assumed to be 0.1.

This is what we call a statistical hypothesis, also frequently referred to as a *null* hypothesis. The latter mostly refers to a hypothesis of an effect measure being neutral, i.e. the parameter being equal to some null (neutral) value.

Quantifying the evidence against the hypothesis is basically computing the probability of getting a body of data less compatible with the hypothesis than the actually observed data, assuming that the hypothesis is true. This probability is known as the p-value for the hypothesis. A convention has been established to 'reject' the null hypothesis if the p-value is small, usually less than 5%. The rationale is that if there is only a very small probability of observing data less compatible with the null hypothesis than the observed data, then the observed data are presumably not compatible with the null hypothesis. In other words, if we observe data that are far away from what the hypothesis predicts, it is likely that it is the hypothesis that is wrong, not the observed data.

The practical calculation of the p-value as the probability of a more extreme result relies on some measure of the distance from the hypothesis to the data and some version of the central limit theorem mentioned in section 3.1.4. Usually we assume that the estimate of our parameter approximately follows a normal distribution with mean as postulated in the hypothesis (in our example a prevalence of 10%), and standard error as derived from the likelihood function.

This has the consequence that we can devise a test for a hypothesis of whether a parameter β (in our example the theoretical prevalence, π) is equal to some null value

β_0 (in our example 10%). This is done by using the distributional assumptions of the estimator $\hat{\beta}$, whereby $(\hat{\beta} - \beta_0)/\text{s.e.}(\beta)$ (the *test statistic*) will approximately follow a normal distribution with mean 0 and standard deviation 1 if the hypothesis $\beta = \beta_0$ is true. The p-value is then defined as the probability of getting a test statistic that is numerically larger than the observed test statistic, assuming the hypothesis is true. The only aspect of the assumption we use is that if the hypothesis is true then the test-statistic is a random draw from the standard normal distribution.

The practical calculation in the case of the theoretical prevalence uses the estimate and the standard error as derived:

$$\hat{\pi} = 16/100 = 0.0160, \qquad \text{s.e.}(\hat{\pi}) = \sqrt{\pi(1-\pi)/n} = 0.0367$$

There is a little bit of cheating here, because the standard error of $\hat{\pi}$ depends on π—which we do not know—so we have bluntly inserted $\hat{\pi}$ for π in the formula for the standard error.

```
> n <- 100
> p <- 16 / n
> ( se.p <- sqrt( p * (1-p) / n) )
[1] 0.03666061
> tt.p <- ( p - 0.1 ) / se.p
> 2 * pnorm( abs(tt.p), lower.tail = FALSE )
[1] 0.1017069
```

CODE EXPLAINED: `p` is the empirical prevalence, the estimate; `se.p` is the standard error of it; `tt.p` is the test statistic measuring the distance to the hypothesis of $\pi = 0.1$. `abs` computes the the absolute value of this, and `pnorm` with the argument `lower.tail=FALSE` returns the probability of a normal random variate being larger than the value of the first argument (`abs(tt.p)`). We want to see what the probability of a larger deviation from 0.1 than the one observed is in *either direction*. But we only computed it in one direction so we must multiply by 2 to get the probability of seeing a more extreme value in either direction.

The simple hand-calculation returns a p-value of 0.102. From a traditional point of view this is non-significant, and we conclude that there is no evidence against the (null) hypothesis of a theoretical prevalence of diabetes of 10%.

A variant of this is done on the log-scale using the modelling—the hypothesis is then changed from $\pi = 0.1$ to $\log(p) = \log(0.1)$:

```
> ml <- glm( cbind(x, n-x) ~ 1, family = binomial(link=log) )
> ci.lin(ml)
            Estimate    StdErr         z          P       2.5%      97.5%
(Intercept) -1.832581 0.2291288 -7.998041 1.264139e-15 -2.281666 -1.383497
> tt.m <- (-1.832581 - log(0.10) ) / 0.2291288
> 2 * pnorm( abs(tt.m), lower.tail=FALSE )
[1] 0.04024106
> Wald( ml, H0=log(0.1) )
    Chisq        d.f.          P
4.20768414 1.00000000 0.04024124
```

CODE EXPLAINED: We fit the model for the log-prevalence using `glm` as on p. 53, `ci.lin` shows the estimates as rendered by `glm`, that is the log-prevalence and the standard error of this computed from the model, and `tt.m` holds the test-statistic using `log(0.1)` as the reference values and the computed standard error of the log-prevalence. The p-value is computed the same way as before.

Note that by default the p-value in the model result is for the hypothesis that the parameter (in this case $\log(\pi)$) is 0, so the hypothesis tested by default is that the prevalence is 1 (100%) (since $\log(1) = 0$). So the default p-value from the default model output is meaningless in this case.

The `Wald` function is a wrapper for `ci.lin` which does the calculation for any null hypothesis (given by the argument `H0`)—the small difference in p-values is because the hand-calculated p-value is based on the estimate and standard error from the `glm` output rounded to (only!) 7 decimals.

We can also do the same calculation on the logit scale:

```
> ml <- glm( cbind(x, n-x) ~ 1, family = binomial )
> ci.lin(ml)
            Estimate    StdErr         z          P       2.5%      97.5%
(Intercept) -1.658228 0.2727724 -6.079165 1.208103e-09 -2.192852 -1.123604
> Wald( ml, H0=logit(0.1) )
    Chisq       d.f.          P
3.90455158 1.00000000 0.04815548
```

CODE EXPLAINED: This is parallel to the previous, except that we use the logit link instead, and so the null value supplied to Wald must be the logit of 0.1, and not the log of 0.1.

So we see that using the normal approximation to the distribution of $\log(\hat\pi)$ rather than that of $\hat\pi$ gives a p-value for the hypothesis of 0.040 instead of 0.102, and when using the logit a p-value of 0.048. These p-values are not dramatically different, but adherers to the religion of the 5% significance level will draw different conclusions depending on what transformation is chosen. Using the log-scale will make them conclude that the observed prevalence is not compatible with a theoretical prevalence of 10%; using the prevalence-scale will make them conclude that it is. Using the logit scale may leave them undecided. Unfortunately, there is nothing in the scriptures that provides guidance as to which scale to use.

The two confidence intervals are, as we saw above, based on the prevalence scale $(8.8, 23.3)$% and based on the log-prevalence scale $(10.2, 25.1)$%, so largely uninformative in the sense that 16 out of 100 is compatible with theoretical prevalences in the range 10 to 24%. Whether 10% is formally in that range seems to be a pretty moot question. It is not reasonable to conclude anything based on a p-value. Ever.

Sometimes the conclusion is that too little information is available to draw any conclusion.

3.2 Prevalence by age

Of course we will not be content with just having an estimate of the prevalence of diabetes among 60-year-old men; we would like to know what the prevalence is at *any* age and naturally also separately for men and women. So we want to expand the model to all ages and also to both sexes.

We will use the *total* data in `pr`, so in the interpretation we will not include the sampling variation; some would claim there is then no variation left because we (in principle at least) classified the entire population as diabetic or not. What we are after is a description of a probability machinery that *could* have generated the data at hand—it is characteristics of this machinery that will tell us about relevant features of the prevalence of diabetes. Note that there may be (many, perhaps) other conceivable machineries that could have generated data. What we will do is to impose a structure on the probability model that allows us to extract characteristics about the diabetes prevalence that we are interested in.

The dataset `pr` has the number of diabetes patients and the population size as of 2010-01-01 in 1-year intervals, so we can compute the *empirical* prevalences by age and sex (but only print some of them):

```
> prt <- stat.table( index = list(A, sex),
+                    contents = ratio(X, N, 100), data = pr )[1,,]
> round( prt[70:75,], 1 )
    sex
A       M    F
  69 16.2 12.4
  70 16.5 12.7
  71 17.3 13.5
  72 17.7 13.9
  73 18.3 14.8
  74 18.9 15.1
```

> CODE EXPLAINED: `stat.table` makes a table classified by the variables listed in the `index` argument. Each cell has a content as specified by the `contents` argument, in this case the ratio of X to N. In this case we get a two-way array classified by age and sex, with the ratio X/N (multiplied by 100) in each cell. A few rows of the resulting array is printed using the indexing facility; `[70:75,]` selects *rows* 70 through 75, because `70:75` is before the comma.
>
> Note the 70th row of the table is that with age-class 69; this is because row number 1 is age-class 0.

We can plot these entries as a function of age, with one curve for each sex:

```
> matplot( 0:99+0.5, prt, type="l", lwd=2, col=c(4,2), lty=1 )
> abline( v=c(76,81)+0.5)
```

> CODE EXPLAINED: The first argument to `matplot` is the vector of (common) *x*-values for the two curves. `prt` is a two-column table, so each column is plotted versus `0:99+0.5`. The `abline` function adds straight lines to the plot; using the `v=` argument gives vertical lines, here at ages 76 and 81 to illustrate the ages of maximal prevalences for men and women. We plotted the prevalences against the midpoints of the age-classes, so we add 0.5 to the position of the vertical lines too (Figure 3.1).

The overall patterns are pretty clear; a peak around 76 for men and around 81 for women, but the curves seem quite erratic, particularly towards the end. Some may argue that these *are* the prevalences, and further modelling is superfluous.

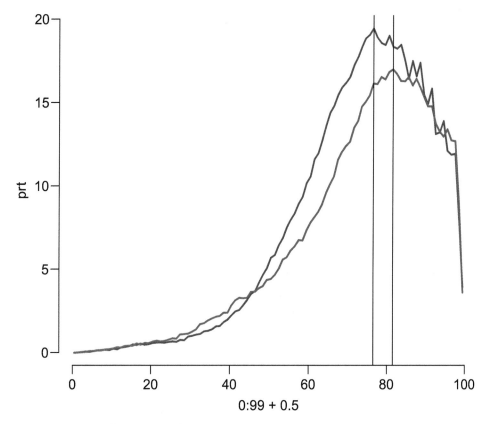

Figure 3.1 Empirical prevalence of diabetes in Denmark 2010 by age—midpoint ages connected by lines.

But a modelling approach allows us to estimate how the prevalence varies by age under an assumption that it does so smoothly. The assumption is that there is some 'true' probability of being a diabetes patient and that this varies smoothly by age. What we observe in *data* in the chosen age-classes is a combination of the smoothly varying true prevalence and random fluctuations in the population.

We fit a smooth model separately for men and and women for the age-specific prevalences using what is known as a natural spline implemented by Ns in the Epi package—this is not elaborated here; a more extensive description is given in Chapter 6 on parametrization. Note that we add 0.5 to A because the average age in the age-group 67, say, is approximately 67.5 years:

```
> pr$A <- pr$A+0.5
> ma <- glm( cbind(X,N-X) ~ Ns( A, knots=c(10,30,50,60,70,80,90) ),
+            family = binomial,
+               data = subset(pr, sex=="M") )
> fa <- glm( cbind(X,N-X) ~ Ns( A, knots=c(10,30,50,60,70,80,90) ),
+            family = binomial,
+               data = subset(pr, sex=="F") )
> fa <- update( ma, data = subset(pr, sex=="F") )
```

The binomial response must be a two-column matrix (cbind, binds vectors as columns together to a matrix), where the first column (X) contains counts of the diabetes patients, and the second column (N-X) the counts of the non-affected persons in the population. Note that the response columns must be (events,non-events), *not* (events,total). The probability is modelled as a smooth function of age (A), here a natural spline (Ns()) which produces a piece-wise cubic function—it is cubic between the knots, linear before the first and after the last knot, and nicely fitted together *at* the knots.

The model statements for men and women are identical; the only difference is the data argument that via subset selects different subsets of the data frame for the analysis. The second statement producing the object fa gives the same result as the first; the update function fits the same model as ma, *except* for the arguments given. For further details about update see p. 62.

Once we have fitted the models we can make predictions of the prevalences for men and women, and because we have a continuous, smooth model, we can make the predictions at *any* age, not only for those in the dataset. Formally, we are modelling discrete (grouped) data—counts in 1-year classes, but we have attached a *quantitative* score to each class as the basis for estimating a continuous relationship between age and prevalence of diabetes. A truly quantitative model would require that we had a dataset with the diabetes status (yes/no) and the exact age of each person in the entire population as of 2010-01-01.

In order to show this quantitative relationship we use a prediction data frame with variables named as the explanatory variables in the model (in this case only A):

```
> matplot( 0:99, prt, yaxs="i", ylim=c(0,20),
+         xlab="Age", ylab="Prevalence of diabetes 2010 (%)",
+         type="s", lwd=1, col=c("blue","red"), lty=1 )
> nd <- data.frame( A=seq(0,100,0.2) )
> pr.m <- ci.pred( ma, nd ) * 100
> pr.f <- ci.pred( fa, nd ) * 100
> matshade( nd$A, cbind(pr.m,pr.f), col=c("blue","red"), lwd=1, alpha=0.2 )
```

matplot plots one curve for each column in prt—the two-column matrix of empirical prevalences for men, respectively women, in 1-year intervals, against the vector 0:99, the age-class. The specification type="s" produces a step function where the points are at the left side of the steps, so that we, for example, for age-class 42 get a small horizontal line stretching from 42 to 43, at the level of the prevalence of a 42 year old. The yaxs="i" requires the *y*-axis to be precisely from 0 to 20; normally ylim=c(0,20) would give a *y*-axis from a bit below 0 to a bit above 20. Since the quantity plotted (prevalence) is necessarily positive (well, non-negative), this should be reflected in the graph, so the *y*-axis should not extend below 0.

The data frame nd ('newdata') has a column for each of the covariates in the model, with values for which we want predictions—in this case the only covariate is age (A) from 0 to 100 in steps of 0.2 years. ci.pred makes predictions from the models (ma and fa), at the points indicated in nd. Each row in nd represents an age at which we want a prediction of prevalence.

The function matshade plots curves (on top of an existing plot) with confidence intervals shown as shaded areas. The first argument to matshade is the *x*-variable;

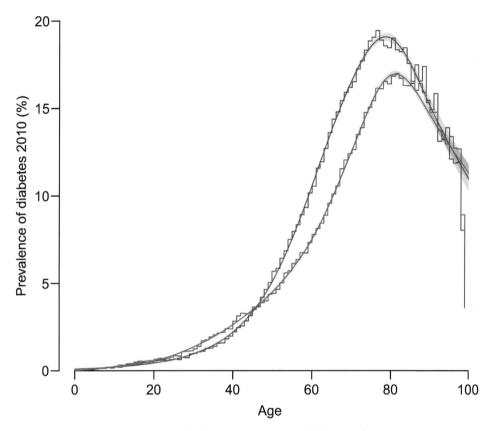

Figure 3.2 Empirical prevalence of diabetes in Denmark 2010 (step function) and estimated (theoretical) prevalence with 95% confidence intervals as shades. Blue is men; red is women.

the second is the *y*-variable(s) with confidence limits, which is expected to be a matrix with 3 columns (estimate,lower,upper) per curve, in this case 6 columns in `cbind(pr.m,pr.f)`.

The *empirical* prevalences are illustrated by the step function; they are tied to a particular grouping of the data; for example, by sex and/or age class. Using the *theoretical* prevalences based on the *modelling* we can refer to *any* combination of sex and age; after modelling we can in principle refer to the prevalence of diabetes in women aged 68.3 years or men aged 73.6 years, because we regard the prevalence as a continuous function of age (Figure 3.2).

If we were to make any statements about the age dependence of the prevalence of diabetes in Denmark in 2010, it is the latter we would use as basis. It is common sense that the prevalence of diabetes varies continuously smoothly with age and not in steps, which of course should be reflected in the modelling and reporting of prevalences. The estimated prevalences we refer to are *theoretical* prevalences—what is the probability that a randomly chosen man of a given age, say 73.6 years has diabetes? The confidence intervals are confidence intervals for these probabilities.

3.3 Comparing different models for the same data

When we chose the knots for the splines to model the age-effect on prevalence, the knots were more or less taken out of thin air. A reasonable question would be if we could get away with using fewer knots, say 10, 50, 70, and 90? Or if we would get a substantial improvement of the model fit by adding knots at 65 and 75?

Thus we want to compare different models for the same data, models that describe data in various degrees of detail. Note in the examples we deliberately chose models that were *nested*, in the sense that one model could be obtained from another by adding or deleting knots in the description of the age-effect.

3.3.1 *Likelihood-ratio test*

It is possible to compare a given model with a simpler model using what is called the likelihood-ratio test. This is based on the property that the ratio of the likelihoods for two models (on the assumption that the simpler of the models is the correct one) has a known distribution. If the simplest model is the 'true' model, then fitting a more elaborate model should add nothing, and by that token the difference between the two model fits is random noise, and some suitable transformation of that will follow some null distribution. So if we get a difference between models that is not compatible with the null distribution we conclude that there actually *is* an improvement by using the more elaborate model.

It should be stressed that 'a simpler model' means a model which is *nested* in the given model in the sense that the simpler can be obtained from the given model by removing some of the parameters.

It can be shown that twice the difference in log-likelihoods between a true model and an (unnecessary) extension of it follows a χ^2-distribution (chi-squared distribution). The χ^2-distribution comes in different shapes, indexed by the *degrees of freedom*. The number of degrees of freedom to be used when comparing two models is the difference in the number of *parameters* in the models.

So if we try to fit the simplification and extension of the prevalence model above we can ask R to compute the differences in log-likelihood between the models. What is actually computed is what we call the *deviance* for each model and subsequently the differences between these.

3.3.2 *Deviance*

A *saturated* model for a given dataset is a model with one parameter per record in the dataset. This will normally not be a model that has any particular interest—it will have way too many parameters.

The likelihood-ratio test statistic of a particular model versus the saturated model is called the deviance (sometimes the *residual* deviance). This is easier to compute than the log-likelihood, so this is what R provides for (almost) all models.

The deviance is associated with a number of degrees of freedom equal to the number of observations in the dataset minus the number of parameters in the model. Or more precisely, it is the difference in the number of fitted parameters in the saturated model and in the model of interest.

If we want to test whether a particular model for a given dataset gives a better description than another, we can compare deviances instead of log-likelihoods—the difference in deviances will be the same as the difference in (twice) the log-likelihoods, because the

saturated full model used in the calculation is the same in the two deviances. This is what
is done with the anova command:

```
> m1 <- glm( cbind(X,N-X) ~ Ns( A, knots=c(10,    50,        70,        90) ),
+              family = binomial, data = subset(pr,sex=="M") )
> m2 <- glm( cbind(X,N-X) ~ Ns( A, knots=c(10,30,50,60,    70,    80,90) ),
+              family = binomial, data = subset(pr,sex=="M") )
> m3 <- glm( cbind(X,N-X) ~ Ns( A, knots=c(10,30,50,60,65,70,75,80,90) ),
+              family = binomial, data = subset(pr,sex=="M") )
> anova( m1, m2, m3, test="Chisq" )
Analysis of Deviance Table

Model 1: cbind(X, N - X) ~ Ns(A, knots = c(10, 50, 70, 90))
Model 2: cbind(X, N - X) ~ Ns(A, knots = c(10, 30, 50, 60, 70, 80, 90))
Model 3: cbind(X, N - X) ~ Ns(A, knots = c(10, 30, 50, 60, 65, 70, 75,
    80, 90))
  Resid. Df Resid. Dev Df Deviance  Pr(>Chi)
1        96     521.30
2        93     458.80  3   62.501 1.717e-13
3        91     456.84  2    1.953   0.3767
```

> CODE EXPLAINED: The three glm models fitted for the prevalence of diabetes among Danish
> men only differ in the number and position of knots in the chosen splines that describe
> the age-effect. The anova function compares the three models successively by evaluating
> the deviances and the successive differences between these.

From the output we see that from a purely p-value point of view, model m2 represents a
substantial improvement of fit over the model m1, while m3 does not represent any further
improvement. Thus if only these three models are considered would we report results from
the model m2.

3.3.3 Deviance and goodness of fit

Sometimes the deviance is used as a χ^2-statistic with its degrees of freedom as a test of
'goodness of fit'. Formally, this is a test of the fitted model against the model with one
parameter per data unit.

First, this depends strongly on the shape of the dataset—if we had obtained the
prevalence data in 2-year age-classes, it would mean that the saturated model would be
different from the one we used based on the 1-year age-classes.

Second, the deviance provides a very unspecific test—the larger model is the saturated
model, but the adequacy of a model is better assessed by testing the model against a model
representing specific extension, e.g. inclusion of an interaction between two variables that
will make sense from a subject-matter point of view.

From a glm it is possible to extract the deviance (deviance) and its degrees of freedom
(df.residual), as well as the *null* deviance (null.deviance)—the deviance of the
model with only an intercept and the corresponding degrees of freedom (df.null) (which
will always be one less than the number of rows in the dataset).

```
> c( m1$deviance, m1$null.deviance )
[1]    521.2969 192538.6812
> c( nrow(m1$data), m1$df.residual, m1$df.null )
[1] 100  96  99
```

If the model is specified without an intercept the null deviance will be the deviance of a model with a linear predictor of 0:

```
> m0 <- update( m1, . ~ . -1 )
> c( m0$deviance, m0$null.deviance )
[1] 1124383 2883984
> c( nrow(m0$data), m0$df.residual, m0$df.null )
[1] 100  97 100
```

> CODE EXPLAINED: The update function also makes it possible to change the response variable and the model for the predictors, using '.' to refer to the response and predictor parts of the model (m1), so that . -1 means the predictor used in m1 with a -1 added— that is, the model with the intercept removed.
> We see that when the intercept is removed, the null deviance has 100 d.f. equal to the number of records in the dataset, because we are comparing to the model without any parameters, i.e. a linear predictor equal to 0 corresponding to $\text{logit}(\pi) = 0 \Leftrightarrow \pi = 0.5$. Not a very sensible model it should be noted.

3.3.4 AIC and BIC

Aikaike's Information Criterion (AIC) is a quantity computed for a set of models fitted to the *same* set of data. It is designed to measure the information loss relative to some supposedly unknown true model. The smaller the criterion is, the better the fit of the model to the dataset at hand. It basically consists of minus twice the log-likelihood (which is smaller for a better model fit), adding twice the number of parameters as a penalty for using a lot of parameters to obtain a good fit. The criterion thus balances model fit and number of parameters in the model. When comparing the AIC between different models one would normally choose the one with the smallest value of AIC.

The AIC is computed by glm, it is printed by the summary command, and it can also be found in the aic element of the model list:

```
> summary(m1)
Call:
glm(formula = cbind(X, N - X) ~ Ns(A, knots = c(10, 50, 70, 90)),
    family = binomial, data = subset(pr, sex == "M"))

Deviance Residuals:
    Min      1Q   Median      3Q      Max
-7.6946  -1.6064  -0.3651   1.5409   6.0615

Coefficients:
                                   Estimate Std. Error z value Pr(>|z|)
(Intercept)                        -6.22959    0.02229  -279.5   <2e-16
Ns(A, knots = c(10, 50, 70, 90))1   4.22055    0.01541   273.9   <2e-16
Ns(A, knots = c(10, 50, 70, 90))2   7.04255    0.04869   144.6   <2e-16
Ns(A, knots = c(10, 50, 70, 90))3   3.01622    0.01377   219.0   <2e-16

(Dispersion parameter for binomial family taken to be 1)

    Null deviance: 192538.7  on 99  degrees of freedom
```

```
Residual deviance:      521.3  on 96  degrees of freedom
AIC: 1326.7

Number of Fisher Scoring iterations: 4
> c( m1$aic, m2$aic, m3$aic )
[1] 1326.683 1270.183 1272.230
```

From the output we see that m2 has the smaller AIC; m1 was by the likelihood-ratio test substantially worse fitting, while m3 did not provide any better fit despite more parameters. So also by the AIC we would have chosen the model m2.

The Bayesian information criterion is another measure of model fit, but built on a different basis, so the penalty is not twice the number of parameters but the number of parameters multiplied by the log of the number of observations in data.

Comparative studies are ambiguous as to which is the better criterion, but there are indications that AIC is better than BIC in finite samples—which is what is normally considered in practice. BIC is not routinely computed in summaries of glm models, but the stats4 package has a function BIC that will compute the BIC from a glm model:

```
> library( stats4 )
> c( BIC(m1), BIC(m2), BIC(m3) )
[1] 1337.104 1288.419 1295.676
```

From this we see that we would reach the same conclusion as before.

CHAPTER 4

Regression models

This chapter is meant as a reference chapter on how to code and interpret the effect of covariates in regression models. To this end we will use the standard normal linear model.

4.1 Types of models

There are four main types of response variables in probability models:

- quantitative (or metric): a measurement of, say, a person's height, blood pressure, annual income. A quantitative variable can in principle take any numerical value; from a modelling perspective this includes negative values, even if most quantitative variables encountered only can assume positive values.

  The appropriate model for this type of response is the normal linear model, assuming that the *mean* of the response depends on the explanatory variables via a linear function. This is what we will introduce in this chapter to illustrate general features of models.
- binary: classification of the presence or absence of some condition—typically the presence of a particular disease as we saw in Chapter 3 on the prevalence of diabetes. In practical modelling the response can be either a two-column matrix of successes and failures or a vector of 0s and 1s.

  The appropriate model for this type of response is a *binomial regression* model, where some function (such as the log-odds) of the probability depends on the explanatory variables via a linear function; see Chapters 3 and 7.
- count: counts of the number of persons or items; we saw the count of (prospective) students of UCLB classified by various factors. A special case of this is aggregated binary data.

  The appropriate model for this type of response is a *Poisson model* for the counts. Special cases of this coincides with certain types of binomial regression models; but this is not detailed in this book.
- rate: recordings of follow-up in the form of events and follow-up time. This type of response differs from the other three in that it is *bivariate* in the form of (events,time). Also, rate data may be represented in different degrees of aggregation as we shall see in Chapter 5.

  Appropriate models for this type of response is either a variant of the Poisson model with allowance for the follow-up time or a survival type model such as the Cox model.

  The response variable is either a count (and a corresponding log-risk-time as offset) or a two-column matrix of events and risk time; see Chapter 5.

Epidemiology with R. Bendix Carstensen, Oxford University Press (2021). © Bendix Carstensen.
DOI: 10.1093/oso/9780198841326.003.0005

- survival: time survived, at the end of which the person is either alive ('censored') or dead. This is not really a fifth type of model; it is merely a type of follow-up study where all persons start at time 0.

  Appropriate models for this type of outcome are as for a rate model. The response is bivariate; the survival time and the event status. In clinical studies, the response will normally be a `Surv` object; see Chapter 8.

A logistic regression model was introduced in Chapter 3 without much explanation of the coding of the covariate age. This and Chapter 5 explains the coding of covariates more thoroughly using linear regression and generalized linear regression models as examples.

4.2 Normal linear regression model

The word 'normal' here refers to the normal probability distribution (also called the Gaussian distribution) which is the distribution assumed for the response variable (conditional on the explanatory variables).

The normal linear regression model establishes a relationship between a quantitative response (also called outcome or dependent) variable, assumed to be normally distributed, and one or more explanatory (also called regression, predictor, or *in*dependent) variables about which *no* distributional assumptions are made. The model is usually referred to as 'the general linear model'.

The response variable is usually termed y, and the explanatory variables x_1, x_2, x_3, etc. The data modelled are observations (measurements) of the variables on a set of persons (or mice or Petri dishes or trees or ...), indexed by i, say:

$$y_i, x_{1i}, x_{2i}, x_{3i}, \dots, \qquad i = 1, \dots, I$$

The data can be arranged in a rectangular data frame (as it is called in R-lingo) with y and the *x*es as columns (in this case 1+3=4) and each person as a row—normally with many more rows than columns.

As an example, the `diet` data frame in the `Epi` package has data on dietary intake, various clinical measurements, and follow-up for coronary heart disease on 337 persons (type `?diet` to see a complete description). We illustrate the relationships of weight, height, energy, fat, and occupation for a start:

```
> library( Epi )
> data( diet )
> head( diet[,c("weight","height","energy","fat","job")] )
    weight  height  energy    fat         job
1 88.17984 181.610 22.8601  9.168       Driver
2 58.74120 165.989 23.8841  9.651       Driver
3 49.89600 152.400 24.9537 11.249    Conductor
4 89.40456 171.196 22.2383  7.578       Driver
5 97.07040 177.800 18.5402  9.147  Bank worker
6 61.00920 175.260 20.3073  8.536  Bank worker
```

CODE EXPLAINED: The `data` function loads the `diet` data. `head` lists the first 6 rows of the dataset; in this case we selected five columns by indexing with `[,]` where the position *after* the comma refers to columns of the data frame, in this case indexed by a character vector of the variable names.

```
> with( diet, plot( weight ~ height, pch=16, cex=0.8,
+                   xlab="Height (cm)", ylab="Weight (kg)" ) )
```

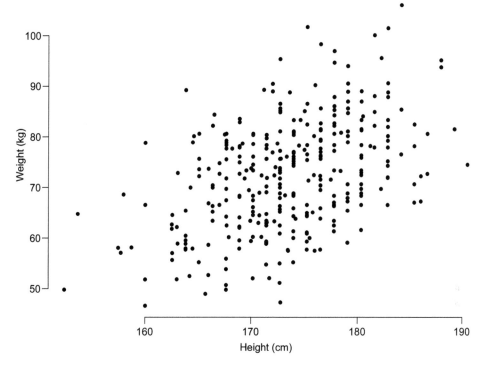

Figure 4.1 Weight versus height in the `diet` dataset. There seems to be a positive relation—tall people weigh more than short people, hardly a surprise.

> CODE EXPLAINED: `with` is a function that allows the code to refer to variables in a data frame (in this case `diet`), so as to avoid writing `diet$weight`, etc.
>
> We used the tilde (~) notation of the plot variables where the *y*-variable is on the left-hand side of the tilde and the *x*-variable on the right-hand side; alternatively, we could have written `plot(height,weight)`. The `pch=16` selects plotting symbol no. 16, which is a circular blob, and `cex=0.8` makes the symbol 80% the default size. The resulting plot is in Figure 4.1.

4.3 Simple linear regression

The term 'simple linear regression' covers the regression model where there is one response variable and one explanatory variable, assuming a linear relationship between the two.

The linear model states that the response *y* is generated as a linear combination of the *x*es plus a random error, e_i:

$$y_i = \beta_0 + \beta_1 x_{1i} + e_i$$

The e_is are assumed to be normally distributed variates that are *independent* with mean 0 and a common variance σ^2. It is the distributional assumption about the e_is that induces the normal distribution of the response variable. Note that there are *no* distributional assumptions about the explanatory variable *x*. Formally this is because the model is a model for the *conditional* distribution of *y* given *x*.

This model has three parameters describing the relationship:

- 2 mean-value parameters, describing the *systematic* variation of y as function of x:
  - β_0—the intercept parameter, the mean (expectation) of y for observations where x is 0. This implies that β_0 is measured in the same units as y.
  - β_1—the effect of x on the response. β_1 is the expected difference in y-values between persons that differ 1 in the value of x_1.

    Since the effect has the form $\beta_1 x_{1i}$ and since this term must have the same dimension as y, it follows that β_1 is measured in units of y per x_1. So if y is weight measured in kg and x_1 is height measured in cm, then β_1 is measured in kg/cm, that is, how many kg does weight increase per cm increase in height. Or more correctly, what is the expected weight difference between two persons that differ 1 cm in height.
- 1 variance parameter, σ^2—usually called the *residual* variance, which estimates the *random* variation of the response, beyond what is explained by x.

    The residuals e_i are assumed to be normally distributed with mean 0 and variance σ^2 which implies that there is 68.3% probability that the observed y is within $\pm 1 \times \sigma$ (note, *not* σ^2) of the predicted and that there is 95.4% probability that the observed y is within $\pm 2 \times \sigma$ of the predicted. This is a consequence of the particular shape of the normal distribution, and thus relies on the distributional assumptions about the residuals (the e_is).

    Note that the relevant parameter therefore is the standard deviation, σ, which is measured in the same units as the response y; σ^2 is rarely interpretable because it is not measured in the same units as y.

4.4 Multiple regression

The general linear model states that the response y (y_i is the value for the ith individual) is generated as a linear combination of the $x$es plus a random error, e_i:

$$y_i = \beta_0 + \beta_1 x_{1i} + \beta_2 x_{2i} + \beta_3 x_{3i} + e_i$$

The e_is are assumed to be normally distributed variates that are *independent* with a common variance σ^2. It is the distributional assumption about the es that induces the normal distribution of the response variable.

Thus the model with 3 independent variables has $5(= 1 + 3 + 1)$ parameters:

- 4 mean-value parameters, describing the *systematic* variation of y as function of the $x$es:
  - β_0—the intercept parameter, the mean (expectation) of y for observations where all $x$es are 0. This implies that β_0 is measured on the same scale as y—it is measured in the same units as y.
  - $\beta_j, j = 1, 2, 3$—the effect of each x on the response. β_j is the expected difference in y-values between persons that differ 1 in the value of x_j but with identical values for all other x-variables.

    Since the effect has the form $\beta_j x_{ji}$ and since this must have the scale as y, it follows that β_j is measured in units of y per x_j. So the β_js are measured in different units if the x_js are.
- 1 variance parameter, σ^2—usually called the *residual* variance, which estimates the *random* variation of the response. Think of this as the part of the variation in y which is not explained by the $x$es. The residuals e_i are assumed to be normally distributed,

which implies that there is 68% probability that the observed y is within $\pm 1 \times \sigma$ (*not* σ^2) of the predicted and that there is 95% probability that the observed y is within $\pm 2 \times \sigma$ of the predicted. This is a consequence of the particular shape of the normal distribution as we just saw above.

4.4.1 *Estimation in the normal linear regression model*

The estimation is done by maximum likelihood, which coincides with the least-squares estimation; the estimates of the βs are the values that minimize $\sum_i (y_i - \beta_0 - \beta_1 x_{1i} - \beta_2 x_{2i} - \beta_3 x_{3i})^2$; hence the name 'least-squares estimation' or 'ordinary least squares' (abbreviated as OLS). The estimates are usually called $\hat{\beta}_0$, etc., using a caret to distinguish estimates from parameters.

If we have n observations, the maximum likelihood estimate of σ^2 is the mean square of the residuals: $\widehat{\sigma^2} = \sum_i (y_i - \hat{\beta}_0 - \hat{\beta}_1 x_{1i} - \hat{\beta}_2 x_{2i} - \hat{\beta}_3 x_{3i})^2 / n$. This is usually corrected by the number of mean-value parameters p (in this example 4) by replacing n with $n - p$. This has the effect that the expected value of the estimate is σ^2—the statistical term for this is that the estimate is *unbiased*, which incidentally means that the expected value of the estimator $\hat{\sigma}$ is not σ. So the estimate of the relevant parameter (σ) is actually biased, but the bias is small and of no practical relevance unless the sample size (n) is very small.

Estimation in a linear regression model is done in R by lm (linear model):

```
> library( Epi )
> data( diet )
> lm( weight ~ height, data=diet )
Call:
lm(formula = weight ~ height, data = diet)

Coefficients:
(Intercept)        height
   -59.9160       0.7642
```

> CODE EXPLAINED: lm fits a linear normal model for the y-variable on the left-hand side of the ~ with the explanatory variable(s) on the right-hand side. The data argument specifies the data frame where the variables mentioned are found.
>
> Writing the function call and not assigning it invokes the print.lm function on the result, which will just print the estimates.

This only gives the the coefficients, but we can get a bit more detail by assigning the result to an R-object and making a summary of this:

```
> m1 <- lm( weight ~ height, data = diet )
> summary( m1 )
Call:
lm(formula = weight ~ height, data = diet)

Residuals:
     Min        1Q    Median        3Q       Max
-24.7361   -7.4553    0.1608    6.9384   27.8130

Coefficients:
             Estimate Std. Error t value Pr(>|t|)
```

```
(Intercept) -59.91601    14.31557   -4.185 3.66e-05
height         0.76421     0.08252    9.261  < 2e-16

Residual standard error: 9.625 on 330 degrees of freedom
  (5 observations deleted due to missingness)
Multiple R-squared:  0.2063,    Adjusted R-squared:  0.2039
F-statistic: 85.76 on 1 and 330 DF,  p-value: < 2.2e-16
```

We see the same estimates as before but also the estimated residual standard error, 9.625. Out of the 337 persons in the `diet` data frame, 5 had missing values for one or more variables in the model, leaving the analysis with 332 observations (n). Since the model has 2 parameters (p) the residual variance has 330 degrees of freedom ($n - p$).

The estimate of the height parameter (0.76421) means that the expected weight difference between two persons that differ 1 cm in weight is 0.76 kg. Or that the effect of height on age is 0.76 kg/cm—recall that the units of the regression parameters (βs) is always in units of response *per* unit of covariate.

The intercept is used in computing the *predicted* weight of a person from the person's height, so if a person is 171 cm tall, the predicted weight of the person is $-59.916 + 0.764 \times 171 = 70.765$ kg

The residual s.d. expresses the variation (between persons) in weight for a given height— here we use the normal distribution assumption—68% of persons with height 171 cm will have a weight within ± 1 s.d. of the mean—that is, within $70.76 \pm 9.625 = (61.14, 80.39)$. Similarly, 95% of the persons with height will have weight within $70.76 \pm 2 \times 9.625 = (51.52, 90.01)$.

This is, however, not quite true, because we have not taken into account the uncertainty in the parameters β_0 (`Intercept`) and β_1 (`height`). We return to this later—the main message is that the residual s.d. is a measure of the variation *between* persons after correcting for the effects of the regression variables.

4.4.2 R-squared

The quantity labelled `R-squared` in the output from `summary(lm)` is frequently referred to as 'percentage variation explained'; indeed it is the difference between the total variance of the response variable (`weight`) and the residual variance, *relative* to the total variance:

```
> ( var(diet$weight,na.rm=TRUE)  - summary(m1)$sigma^2 ) /
+    var(diet$weight,na.rm=TRUE)

[1]  0.2026751
```

(This quantity is not exactly the same as the `R-squared`, due to corrections for the number of parameters estimated.)

While the term 'percentage variation explained' sounds deceptively relevant, it rarely is. It is a comparison of the residual variation with the total variation in the response variable. The residual variation is a meaningful quantity that is likely to be generalizable to other assessments of the relationship between height and weight—it measures the likely inaccuracy of a weight prediction based on height only. But the *total* variation in weight is not likely to be generalizable to another population—it depends to a very large extent on the choice of the study population where weight and height are measured.

Bluntly speaking, the R-squared is comparing a meaningful measure (residual variation) to a meaningless one (the total variation), and therefore it becomes meaningless, and so should be avoided. The value of it is easily manipulated; a short description of this is available at http://bendixcarstensen.com/r-sq.pdf.

The R-squared is also equal to the square of the correlation between `weight` and `height`:

```
> cor( diet$weight, diet$height, use="complete.obs" )^2
[1] 0.2062756
```

CODE EXPLAINED: The function `cor` computes the correlation between two variables. If a matrix is supplied as argument, `cor` will return a matrix of correlations between columns of the matrix.

4.4.3 *Multiple regression*

We may ask whether the variables `energy` (total energy intake, in kcal/day divided by 100) and `fibre` (fibre intake, in units of 10 g/day) also have an effect on the weight of the person:

```
> m3 <- lm( weight ~ height + energy + fibre, data = diet )
> summary( m3 )

Call:
lm(formula = weight ~ height + energy + fibre, data = diet)

Residuals:
     Min       1Q   Median       3Q      Max
-20.6563  -7.1461  -0.3391   6.3311  27.6482

Coefficients:
             Estimate Std. Error t value Pr(>|t|)
(Intercept) -56.72231   13.91401  -4.077 5.75e-05
height        0.66542    0.08054   8.261 3.72e-15
energy        0.26420    0.13394   1.972  0.04941
fibre         3.64190    1.06775   3.411  0.00073

Residual standard error: 9.129 on 324 degrees of freedom
  (9 observations deleted due to missingness)
Multiple R-squared:  0.2797,    Adjusted R-squared:  0.273
F-statistic: 41.93 on 3 and 324 DF,  p-value: < 2.2e-16

> round( ci.lin( m3 ), 3 )
             Estimate StdErr      z     P    2.5%   97.5%
(Intercept)  -56.722 13.914 -4.077 0.000 -83.993 -29.451
height         0.665  0.081  8.261 0.000   0.508   0.823
energy         0.264  0.134  1.972 0.049   0.002   0.527
fibre          3.642  1.068  3.411 0.001   1.549   5.735
```

CODE EXPLAINED: The result of the multiple regression is assigned to `m3`, and the `summary` prints the parameters and other summaries, such as the residual standard error.

`ci.lin` extracts only the estimates and computes the confidence limits for the estimated parameters.

We see that the effect of `height` is approximately the same as before, and that the effect of `energy` is 0.264 kg per 100 kcal per day. The effect of `fibre` is 3.642 kg per 10 g fibre intake per day.

The effects estimated are all *isolated* effects in the sense that they are only interpretable as e.g. the effect of varying energy intake assuming the other variables (height and fibre) are at a constant level. So in this case we are looking at the effect of increasing energy intake without increasing the absolute fibre intake, so actually not just eating more, but also eating differently. This type of interpretation should always be remembered, in particular when regression variables are correlated.

4.4.4 *Standardized variables*

Since regression coefficients for different covariates have different units, they are not comparable—you cannot compare apples and oranges. Therefore quantitative regression variables are sometimes scaled by the (study) population standard deviation (dividing x by s.d.(x)), so that the effects are interpretable as effects per population standard deviation of, say, fibre intake or energy intake. This corresponds to multiplying the original regression coefficient by the population standard error of the variable, thus rendering it with the dimension of the response.

Superficially, this will make regression coefficients for different variables comparable in the sense that they will refer to change in the response variable per 1 population standard deviation. However, this refers to the *study* population variation of different variables; hence only the relative importance of the variables *in the current study population* can be assessed this way. There is no guarantee that the relative sizes of the population standard deviations of different variables are constant across populations, so comparing the standardized effects will not necessarily carry over to other study populations. Even if the actual effects were the same, this would require that the relative sizes of the population variation of the variables be the same in another study population.

So while the phrase 'per population standard deviation' sounds catchy and generalizable, it is often overlooked that 'population' is a shorthand for 'this particular study sample', which is not quite so catchy and certainly not generalizable.

The practicalities of fitting a model with standardized variables is straightforward:

```
> m4 <- lm( weight ~ I(height/sd(height,na.rm=TRUE)) +
+                    I(energy/sd(energy,na.rm=TRUE)) +
+                    I(fibre /sd(fibre ,na.rm=TRUE)),
+            data = diet )
> summary(m4)

Call:
lm(formula = weight ~ I(height/sd(height, na.rm = TRUE)) +
    I(energy/sd(energy, na.rm = TRUE)) +
    I(fibre/sd(fibre, na.rm = TRUE)), data = diet)

Residuals:
     Min      1Q  Median      3Q     Max
-20.6563 -7.1461 -0.3391  6.3311 27.6482

Coefficients:
                                Estimate Std. Error t value Pr(>|t|)
(Intercept)                     -56.7223    13.9140  -4.077 5.75e-05
```

```
I(height/sd(height, na.rm = TRUE))    4.2657    0.5163   8.261 3.72e-15
I(energy/sd(energy, na.rm = TRUE))    1.1671    0.5917   1.972  0.04941
I(fibre/sd(fibre, na.rm = TRUE))      2.0480    0.6004   3.411  0.00073

Residual standard error: 9.129 on 324 degrees of freedom
  (9 observations deleted due to missingness)
Multiple R-squared:  0.2797,    Adjusted R-squared:  0.273
F-statistic: 41.93 on 3 and 324 DF,  p-value: < 2.2e-16
```

> CODE EXPLAINED: We just replace the variables by an expression of the variable divided by its standard deviation. Note that we must include na.rm=TRUE, otherwise the function sd returns NA if the argument has just one missing value.
>
> Comparing the summaries of the model m4 and the previous m3 shows that the intercepts are the same, and the columns t value and Pr(>|t|) are the same because the only thing that has been done is a rescaling of the regression variables.

4.4.5 Predictions from the normal regression model

We can predict a person's weight from a specific set of values of the explanatory variables; the way to go about this is to set up a *prediction data frame*, a data frame with one record per combination of covariate values for which we want a prediction. For a given set of covariate values we can either produce *confidence intervals* for the *mean* response or *prediction intervals* for future observations. The latter will always be wider then the former; they are intervals that capture future observations from the model with a given probability (usually 90 or 95%):

```
> nd <- data.frame( height = c(151:190,NA,150:189),
+                   fibre = rep(c(0.6,2.5),c(40,41)),
+                   energy = 28 )
```

> CODE EXPLAINED: The data frame nd is created to contain combinations of height over the relevant range with two values of fibre and one fixed value of energy. This will give two estimated regression lines. To distinguish these we use heights from 151 to 190 for one and from 150 to 189 for the other. We separate them by an NA, in order to prevent connecting the ends of the lines when plotting. An NA in (one of) the predictor variable(s) will create an NA in the prediction. rep repeats each of the elements of the first argument (c(0.6,2.5)) as many times as given by the second argument (c(40,41)), so 40 times 0.6 follows by 41 times 2.5. The value of energy is automatically repeated to match the 81 rows in the data frame.

```
> pr.m <- predict( m3, interval="conf", newdata=nd )
> pr.p <- predict( m3, interval="pred", newdata=nd )
```

> CODE EXPLAINED: The predict (really predict.lm, because m3 is an lm object) provides predicted values from the model: the first one with confidence intervals of the mean, and the second with prediction intervals for future observations. Both pr.m and pr.p are 3-column structures with estimates in the first column and lower and upper limits of the intervals in the two last.

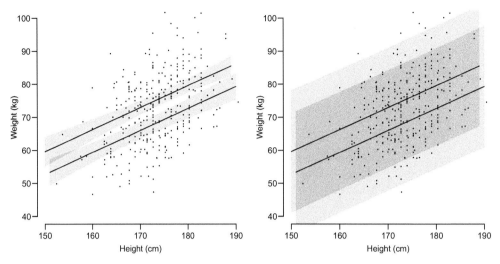

Figure 4.2 Predicted values from a multiple regression model. (Left) The *confidence* intervals for the mean as shaded areas. The lines are for an energy intake of 28 kcal per day/100 and fibre intake of 0.6 (lowest) and 2.5 (highest). (Right) The *prediction* intervals for new observations.

```
> par( mfrow=c(1,2) )
> matshade( nd$height, pr.m, plot=TRUE, ylim=c(40,100),
+          xlab="Height (cm)", ylab="Weight (kg)" )
> with( diet, points( height, weight, cex=0.3, pch=16 ) )
> matshade( nd$height, pr.p, plot=TRUE, ylim=c(40,100),
+          xlab="Height (cm)", ylab="Weight (kg)" )
> with( diet, points( height, weight, cex=0.3, pch=16 ) )
```

CODE EXPLAINED: The argument `mfrow=c(1,2)` sets up the graphical output in a 1 by 2 layout, so that the next two graphs produced will appear side by side. `matshade` produces a plot of the predicted values with a 95% confidence interval (`pr.m`) as a shaded area. `plot=TRUE` tells `matshade` to create a new plot instead of adding to an existing plot, and `ylim` explicitly specifies the extent of the *y*-axis. The latter is necessary if we want the same *y*-axis on both plots. The `with` function allows the function inside (`points`) to refer to columns in the data frame `diet`.

The second call of `matshade` and `points` is a repeat of the first, except that we now plot the *prediction* intervals (`pr.p`).

In Figure 4.2 we see that the prediction intervals are much wider than the confidence intervals for the mean, because they also accommodate the residual variation.

4.5 Model formulae in R

We have used *model formulae* to specify the effects we have in a model. A formula is basically just a '~' with an expression or just a variable on the left and one or more variables or expressions on the right. The left side is the response (outcome, dependent), and it depends on the model; for normal regression it is a quantitative variable, and for binomial regression it is either a binary variable or a two-column matrix of counts, etc.—see p. 65.

Table 4.1 Model formulae in R

`+0`	omit the intercept from the model
`-1`	omit the intercept from the model
`+A`	add term `A` to the model
`-A`	remove term `A` from model
`A:B`	create interaction between `A` and `B`
`A*B`	create main effects and interaction between two terms, equal to `A+B+A:B`
`A/B`	main effect of `A` and interaction between `A` and `B`, equal to `A+A:B`. Commonly called 'B within A'
`(A+B+C)^2`	create main effects and all interactions up to 2nd order between variables, i.e. `A+B+C+A:B+A:C+B:C`
`(A+B+C)^3`	create main effects and all interactions up to 3rd order between variables, i.e. `A+B+C+A:B+A:C+B:C+A:B:C`
`I()`	the `Identity` or `Isolate` function, allowing results of arithmetic expressions to be included in a model; `I(A+B)` will include the sum of variables `A` and `B` in the model.

Note: `A` and `B` are names of variables (quantitative or factors) or terms. This type of model specification is known as the Wilkinson-Rogers notation.

The right hand side of the formula makes it possible to specify effects and interactions via operators such as '+' or ':' which connect variables. These operators look like normal arithmetic operators, but in a model formula they have special meanings, described in Table 4.1. Terms in a model formula can be either single variables or functions that return a variable or a matrix.

Because the operators have special meaning in a model formula, it is not possible to include, for example, the sum of two variables using `A+B`—this will be taken as the main effects of `A` and `B`; if we want to include the sum of `A` and `B` as a variable we must *isolate* it from the model by `Inhibiting` formula interpretation by using `I`, so write `I(A+B)`.

Specifically, if we want to include the square of `A` as a variable we would write `A+I(A^2)`. If you have been using other programs you may be used to creating a separate variable with values equal to `A`-squared and then including this in the model. This is, of course, also possible in R, but it has the drawback that predictions require that the extra variable be supplied in the data frame used to specify predictions. If you use `A+I(A^2)` you only have to supply values of the variable `A` in your prediction data frame.

If you want the effect of the log of `A`, you can just use `log(A)` as part of the formula. You can also supply functions that return a multi-column matrix, in which case each of the columns in the matrix will be taken as an explanatory variable in the model. This was the case when we used `Ns` to describe the age-specific prevalences of diabetes in section 3.2.

4.6 Regression models and generalized linear models

The linear normal model described above is a special variant of a more general class of regression models. In Chapter 3 we saw a statistical model where we described a *binomial* response (prevalence of diabetes) as a function of age.

That was a model for the logit $(\log(1/(1-\pi)))$, where π, the prevalence (a probability), is the response variable and age the explanatory variable.

Later we will consider models for rate data where (the ratio of) two variables (events and person-years) are the relevant response, and where we model the logarithm of the rate as a function of the explanatory variables.

These models are what is commonly termed *generalized* linear models [7]; they are models where some *link* function of (the mean of) the response is a linear function of the explanatory variables. In the case of the binomial model the link was the logit function of the binomial probability π: $\mathrm{link}(\pi) = \mathrm{logit}(\pi) = \log{(\pi/(1-\pi))}$; for the normal linear regression model, the link is the identity function; for a Poisson model used for analysing rates, we normally use the logarithm as a link function.

For any such model we are using a *linear predictor* for the link of the mean. A linear predictor is an expression as we saw for the mean of the weight in the linear regression above. The linear predictor is usually termed η (eta)

$$\eta = \beta_0 + \beta_1 x_{1i} + \beta_2 x_{2i} + \beta_3 x_{3i}$$

In that example the *x*es were merely values of the explanatory variables, but by using transformations of the original variables as *x*es, we will get access to a wider class of models, including models allowing a non-linear effect of the explanatory variable on the response.

In most regression models the default is to include β_0 in the linear predictor; usually termed the intercept (or 'corner', 'grand mean', '%GM' or just '1').

Above we saw the distinction between confidence intervals for the mean and prediction intervals for future observations from the model. Prediction intervals are only relevant in the normal regression model where a special parameter is used to describe the residual variance. In models for proportions (binomial) and rates (Poisson) no such parameter is available.

4.6.1 *Categorical effects*

In the `diet` dataset we have the person's occupation in the categorical variable `job`:

```
> str( diet$job )
 Factor w/ 3 levels "Driver","Conductor",..: 1 1 2 1 3 3 3 3 2 1 ...
> levels( diet$job )
[1] "Driver"      "Conductor"    "Bank worker"
```

> CODE EXPLAINED: The function `str` produces information about the argument, in this case the `job` variable in the `diet` dataset. The `levels` function is used to extract the names of the factor levels—in the correct order.

R recognizes `job` as a categorical variable, normally called a `factor`. If we want to model the mean weight by job category we just enter the variable into the model; it is recognized as a `factor`:

```
> mf <- lm( weight ~ job, data=diet )
> round( ci.lin( mf ), 2 )
                Estimate StdErr    z     P   2.5% 97.5%
(Intercept)        72.96   0.98 74.13 0.00  71.03 74.89
jobConductor       -7.31   1.46 -4.99 0.00 -10.18 -4.44
jobBank worker      3.23   1.28  2.52 0.01   0.72  5.74
```

Table 4.2 Coding of the variables associated with each of the parameters (columns) for persons of each type of job (rows)

Job	(Intercept) β_0	β_D	β_C	β_B	Model formula job	Model formula 0+job
					Linear predictor	
Driver	1	1	0	0	β_0	β_D
Conductor	1	0	1	0	$\beta_0 + \beta_C$	β_C
Bank worker	1	0	0	1	$\beta_0 + \beta_B$	β_B

Note: The standard parametrization is to omit the explanatory variable associated with β_D (the reference level). Using 0+ omits the intercept (explanatory variable associated with β_0) and instead includes the variable associated with the reference level, β_D.

CODE EXPLAINED: The lm function fits a linear model with weight as the response variable and the factor variable job as the explanatory variable.

The function ci.lin just extracts the parameters with estimated standard errors from the model and computes the 95% confidence interval for the parameters (hence the name ci.), and round rounds to two digits after the decimal point.

We see that we get two parameters associated with this labelled by the 2nd and 3rd levels of job. What happened behind the scenes is that R generated what is called indicator variables. These are variables that are equal to 1 for persons with job equal to Conductor, and 0 for all others; and similarly for Bank worker, but not for the first level, Driver.

This is illustrated in Table 4.2: a person whose job is Driver is thus coded 0 for these two variables, so the mean weight of a driver is 72.96 kg—the intercept parameter. The parameters for Conductor and Bank worker are *differences* to the reference level of Driver, so the mean weight of a Conductor is 72.96 + −7.31 = 65.65.

However, we can omit the intercept from the model using the 0+ as a term in the model:

```
> mF <- lm( weight ~ 0 + job, data=diet )
> round( ci.lin( mF ), 2 )
                Estimate StdErr     z P  2.5% 97.5%
jobDriver          72.96   0.98 74.13 0 71.03 74.89
jobConductor       65.65   1.08 60.53 0 63.53 67.78
jobBank worker     76.19   0.82 92.93 0 74.59 77.80
```

Omitting the intercept this way does not change the *model*; it only changes the *parametrization* of the model, so we directly get the mean weight in each job as the parameters. Any predictions from the model will be the same as we get from using in the standard parametrization. The difference between the two parametrizations is illustrated in Table 4.2. In the standard parametrization the intercept (β_0, (Intercept)) is common for all job categories, and so the parameter β_C (jobConductor) refers to the *difference* in weight between conductors and drivers (the reference). In the parametrization without intercept, the β_C refers to the mean weight among conductors.

4.6.2 *Linear and categorical effects*

We may want to take both the job and the height of persons into account when describing the weight of persons:

```
> mm <- lm( weight ~ job + height, data=diet )
> round( ci.lin( mm ), 3 )
                Estimate StdErr      z     P    2.5%   97.5%
(Intercept)      -31.289 15.538 -2.014 0.044 -61.744 -0.835
jobConductor      -5.565  1.406 -3.959 0.000  -8.320 -2.810
jobBank worker     0.697  1.262  0.552 0.581  -1.777  3.171
height             0.605  0.090  6.721 0.000   0.429  0.782
```

We now have a quantitative variable in the model so the intercept will refer to the expected weight of a driver of height 0 cm—note that it is negative. Moreover, we are assuming that the effect of height on weight is the same regardless of occupation, namely 0.605kg/cm. In other words, this is a model that states that the effect of height is the same in all three job categories, but that the absolute level of weight in the three job categories are different, thus a model with 3 different but parallel regression lines describing the dependence of weight on height.

If we want a more manageable parametrization we would want the intercept to refer to a person of height, say, 170 cm (the median height in the dataset is 172 cm)—this is normally called 'centring the variable around 170'.

```
> mM <- lm( weight ~ job + I(height-170), data=diet )
> round( ci.lin( mM ), 3 )
                 Estimate StdErr      z     P    2.5%  97.5%
(Intercept)        71.616  0.947 75.636 0.000 69.761 73.472
jobConductor       -5.565  1.406 -3.959 0.000 -8.320 -2.810
jobBank worker      0.697  1.262  0.552 0.581 -1.777  3.171
I(height - 170)     0.605  0.090  6.721 0.000  0.429  0.782

> anova( mM )
Analysis of Variance Table

Response: weight
                 Df  Sum Sq Mean Sq F value    Pr(>F)
job               2  5906.3  2953.1  33.797 4.511e-14
I(height - 170)   1  3947.1  3947.1  45.173 8.002e-11
Residuals       328 28660.0    87.4
```

The intercept parameter now represents the weight of a driver who is 170 cm tall, while the differences between the occupational groups is still the same. But now the effects of occupation do not represent the differences in means between the occupational groups, but the differences in *conditional* means for any given height, the vertical distance between the regression lines (full lines in Figure 4.3). The parametrization can be illustrated in this table:

	Parametrization
Job	job + I(height-170)
Driver	$\beta_0 \quad\quad + \gamma \times (\text{height} - 170)$
Conductor	$\beta_0 + \beta_C + \gamma \times (\text{height} - 170)$
Bank worker	$\beta_0 + \beta_B + \gamma \times (\text{height} - 170)$

We see that the intercept (β_0) corresponds to the expected weight for a 170 cm tall driver.

4.6.3 *ANOVA–ANCOVA*

In the days of hand calculation a linear model with a categorical variable alone (job, say) was termed an 'analysis of variance' model, abbreviated ANOVA. This comes from the fact that the tests of effects were (and still are) based on calculation and comparison of different variances. Similarly, models with a categorical and a quantitative variable were called 'analysis of covariance', ANCOVA. These terms are still occasionally used, but are mostly found in literature from the past century. You can safely replace these terms by 'general linear model', and not worry further. The function anova performs an old-fashioned ANOVA on a lm object, but the explanation of this is for a history book. Subsequently we shall just use the anova function for comparing different models. The name is just a hint to the good old days.

4.6.4 *Categorical-linear interaction*

We may ask whether it is reasonable to assume that the effect of height is the same in all three job categories. This is asking whether the three lines representing the weight–height relationship for the occupational groups are actually parallel. The simplest way to fit the interaction model is by using the '*'-operator in the model formula:

```
> mi <- lm( weight ~ job*height, data=diet )
> round( ci.lin( mi ), 3 )

                        Estimate StdErr      z     P    2.5%    97.5%
(Intercept)              -77.853 30.588 -2.545 0.011 -137.805 -17.901
jobConductor              51.193 46.205  1.108 0.268  -39.368 141.754
jobBank worker            65.764 37.330  1.762 0.078   -7.402 138.929
height                     0.876  0.178  4.933 0.000    0.528   1.224
jobConductor:height       -0.331  0.271 -1.221 0.222   -0.861   0.200
jobBank worker:height     -0.375  0.215 -1.746 0.081   -0.797   0.046
```

This parametrization is not very useful, and for inspection of parameters it is more useful to use a different one and also centre the height around, say, 170 cm:

```
> mI <- lm( weight ~ 0 + job/I(height-170), data=diet )
> round( ci.lin( mI ), 3 )

                               Estimate StdErr      z     P   2.5%  97.5%
jobDriver                        71.017  1.004 70.711 0.000 69.048 72.985
jobConductor                     66.013  1.033 63.924 0.000 63.989 68.037
jobBank worker                   72.986  1.094 66.740 0.000 70.842 75.129
jobDriver:I(height - 170)         0.876  0.178  4.933 0.000  0.528  1.224
jobConductor:I(height - 170)      0.545  0.204  2.667 0.008  0.145  0.946
jobBank worker:I(height - 170)    0.500  0.121  4.128 0.000  0.263  0.738
```

This way the parameters in the model are the mean weights in each of the three groups conditional on height 170 and the three separate slopes. The precise meanings of the model formula operators ('+', '*', ':', '/', 'I') were explained in section 4.5, and Table 4.1 on p. 75.

The two parametrizations can be illustrated in this table, where γ is the parameter associated with height, and γ_C the parameter for jobConductor:height:

	Parametrization	
Job	`job*height`	`0+job/I(height-170)`
Driver	$\beta_0 \quad\quad + \gamma \times \text{height}$	$\beta_D + \gamma_D \times (\text{height} - 170)$
Conductor	$\beta_0 + \beta_C + \gamma \times \text{height} + \gamma_C \times \text{height}$	$\beta_C + \gamma_C \times (\text{height} - 170)$
Bank worker	$\beta_0 + \beta_B + \gamma \times \text{height} + \gamma_B \times \text{height}$	$\beta_B + \gamma_B \times (\text{height} - 170)$

So using `job*height` we see that the intercept (β_0) corresponds to the expected weight for a 0-cm-tall driver—hence no surprise that it is negative. The effect of height in the reference group (driver) is γ, whereas it is $\gamma + \gamma_C$ among conductors. So in this parametrization γ_C is the *difference* in height effects between conductors and drivers, and β_C is the *difference* in (predicted) weight between a conductor and a driver, both of height 170 cm.

We can compare the main-effects model (parallel lines) with the interaction model (arbitrary lines) with a likelihood-ratio test

```
> anova( mm, mi, test="Chisq" )
Analysis of Variance Table

Model 1: weight ~ job + height
Model 2: weight ~ job * height
  Res.Df   RSS Df Sum of Sq Pr(>Chi)
1    328 28660
2    326 28385  2    274.69   0.2065
```

We see that there is formally little improvement by including the interaction term in the model, but even so it would be useful to see how the interaction looks relative to the main-effects model:

```
> pr1 <- data.frame( height=150:190, job=levels(diet$job)[1] )
> pr2 <- data.frame( height=150:190, job=levels(diet$job)[2] )
> pr3 <- data.frame( height=150:190, job=levels(diet$job)[3] )
```

CODE EXPLAINED: For each of the job categories (`levels(diet$job)[1]`, etc.) we create a prediction data frame (`pr1`, etc.) for heights from 150 through 190 cm. These will be used to generate the predicted weights for each job category in the two different models.

```
> clr <- c("red","blue","forestgreen")
> with( diet, plot( weight ~ height,
+                   pch=16, cex=0.6, col=clr[job],
+                   xlab="Height (cm)", ylab="Weight (kg)" ) )
> matshade( pr1$height, cbind( predict(mm,pr1,i="c"), predict(mi,pr1,i="c"),
+                              predict(mm,pr2,i="c"), predict(mi,pr2,i="c"),
+                              predict(mm,pr3,i="c"), predict(mi,pr3,i="c") ),
+         col=rep(clr,each=2), lty=c("solid","21"), lend="butt",
+         lwd=2, alpha=0.1 )
> text( 155, 105-0:2*3, levels(diet$job), col=clr, font=2, adj=0 )
```

CODE EXPLAINED: When plotting points and lines in different colours, it is useful to put the chosen colours in a vector and refer to this when plotting points, lines, and text; it will then be much easier to change the colours. The plot statement (where all variable names refer to columns in `diet` because it is inside the `with` function) plots the

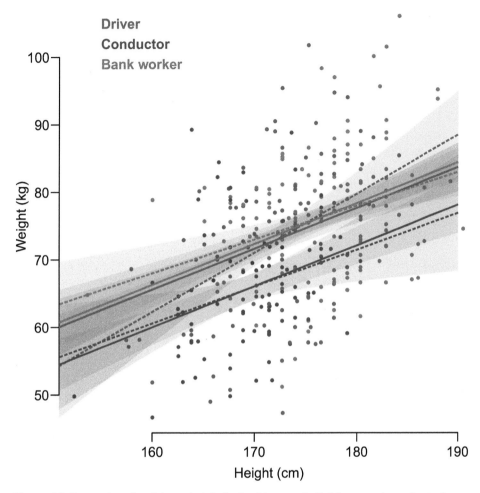

Figure 4.3 Regression of weight on height in the `diet` study. Full lines are the estimated means from the main-effects model (parallel lines); broken lines are estimated means from the interaction model (lines with no restriction).

points with a blob (`pch=16`) of 0.6 times normal size (`cex=0.6`), and in colours from `clr` corresponding to the levels of `job`—indexing ('[ ]') with a factor corresponds to indexing with the *number* of each level.

We make predictions from both the main-effects model (`mm`, which produces 3 parallel lines) and the interaction model (`mi`, which produces 3 lines with no restrictions). The argument `i="c"` to `predict` is really an abbreviation for `interval="confidence"`— an argument name in R can be abbreviated as long as it is unambiguous, and occasionally the value can also be abbreviated.

The predictions are ordered inside the `cbind` by job, then by model, which means that the colours must be repeated twice each (`col=rep(clr,each=2)`) and that the line types must be alternating; the latter is achieved by the recycling rule of R whereby the elements of the vector `c("solid","21")` are repeated as many times as required.

We use the `lty` to define lines; solid lines by (`"solid"`); broken lines `"21"` means two pixels ink, one pixel, none, etc. `lend="butt"` means that the ends of the line pieces that make up the broken line are cut orthogonal to the line; the default is to have the ends rounded. (It is difficult to see, but if you set `lwd=10` or so, the effect will be apparent.)

Special interaction?

We see that the broken lines for `Conductor` and `Bank worker` from the interaction model are almost parallel, so one possible way of looking at an interaction could be to consider a model where these two are assumed to have identical slopes and only `Driver` a different slope.

This type of hypothesis is strongly data-driven, which means that estimates will be biased. Data-driven hypotheses will always provide a too good fit to data, and so should never be entertained. In other words: a model of this type would be sheer nonsense—never embark on that sort of thing even if R have really nice tools to do so very simply.

4.6.5 *Categorical by categorical interaction*

We may ask whether it is reasonable to assume that the effect of the level of energy intake as recorded in the variable `energy.grp` is the same in all job categories:

```
> ma <- lm( weight ~ job + energy.grp, data=diet )
> round( ci.exp( ma, Exp=FALSE ), 3 )

                     Estimate    2.5%   97.5%
(Intercept)            70.554  68.371  72.737
jobConductor           -7.335 -10.134  -4.536
jobBank worker          3.074   0.625   5.523
energy.grp>2750 KCals    4.543   2.451   6.635
```

We see that if we assume that, then high energy intake is associated with a 4.5-kg higher weight.

The question of interactions is quite similar to the categorical–linear interaction treated above, and the syntax of the interaction model looks the same. But the variable is not a quantitative variable, but a `factor` with two levels, `<=2750 KCals` and `>2750 KCals`:

```
> mi <- lm( weight ~ job * energy.grp, data=diet )
> round( ci.lin( mi )[,-3], 3 )
                                     Estimate StdErr     P    2.5%   97.5%
(Intercept)                            71.889  1.394 0.000  69.156  74.622
jobConductor                          -10.442  2.083 0.000 -14.524  -6.361
jobBank worker                          1.817  1.845 0.324  -1.798   5.433
energy.grp>2750 KCals                   2.021  1.916 0.292  -1.735   5.777
jobConductor:energy.grp>2750 KCals      5.831  2.853 0.041   0.239  11.422
jobBank worker:energy.grp>2750 KCals    2.383  2.501 0.341  -2.519   7.285
```

Again, the standard parametrization is not very useful, and for the inspection of parameters it is more useful to use:

```
> mI <- lm( weight ~ 0 + job / energy.grp, data=diet )
> round( ci.lin( mI )[,-3], 3 )
                Estimate StdErr     P    2.5%   97.5%
jobDriver         71.889  1.394 0.000  69.156  74.622
jobConductor      61.447  1.547 0.000  58.415  64.478
jobBank worker    73.706  1.208 0.000  71.340  76.073
```

```
jobDriver:energy.grp>2750 KCals        2.021  1.916 0.292 -1.735  5.777
jobConductor:energy.grp>2750 KCals     7.851  2.113 0.000  3.709 11.994
jobBank worker:energy.grp>2750 KCals   4.404  1.607 0.006  1.254  7.554
```

This way the parameters in the model are the mean weights in each of the three groups in the low energy intake group, and the three separate effects of high energy intake—one for each job category.

The parametrization of the main-effects model and the two different ways of parametrizing the interaction model are illustrated in this table, where δ is the parameter associated with high energy intake, and δ_C the parameter for jobConductor:energy.grp>2750 KCals, etc. Note that the parameters have different values in each model:

Job	Energy	job+energy.grp	job*energy.grp	0+job/energy.grp
			Parametrization	
Driver	Low	β_0	β_0	β_D
Conductor	Low	$\beta_0 + \beta_C$	$\beta_0 + \beta_C$	β_C
Bank worker	Low	$\beta_0 + \beta_B$	$\beta_0 + \beta_B$	β_B
Driver	High	$\beta_0 + \delta$	$\beta_0 + \delta$	$\beta_D + \delta_D$
Conductor	High	$\beta_0 + \beta_C + \delta$	$\beta_0 + \beta_C + \delta + \delta_C$	$\beta_C + \delta_C$
Bank worker	High	$\beta_0 + \beta_B + \delta$	$\beta_0 + \beta_B + \delta + \delta_B$	$\beta_B + \delta_B$

Using the formula job*energy.grp the intercept (β_0) corresponds to the expected weight for a driver with low energy intake. The effect of high energy in the reference group (driver) is δ, whereas it is $\delta + \delta_C$ among conductors. So in this parametrization the δ_C is the *difference* in effects of high energy intake between conductors and drivers, and the β_c is the predicted *difference* in weight between conductors and drivers with a low energy intake.

We can compare the main-effects model (same energy intake effect for all three types of job) with the interaction model with a likelihood-ratio test

```
> anova( ma, mi, test="Chisq" )
Analysis of Variance Table

Model 1: weight ~ job + energy.grp
Model 2: weight ~ job * energy.grp
  Res.Df    RSS Df Sum of Sq Pr(>Chi)
1    329  30906
2    327  30515  2    391.03   0.1231
```

In this case there is little improvement by including the interaction term in the model; the test has 2 degrees of freedom; it is a test of whether $\delta_C = \delta_B = 0$ in the formulation job*energy.grp. If we had used the model formulation job/energy.grp the hypothesis would be $\delta_D = \delta_C = \delta_B$.

4.7 Collinearity and aliasing

It may occur that quantitative variables are strongly correlated; this is, for example, the case for energy and fat in the diet dataset (not really surprising). The phenomenon is occasionally termed collinearity.

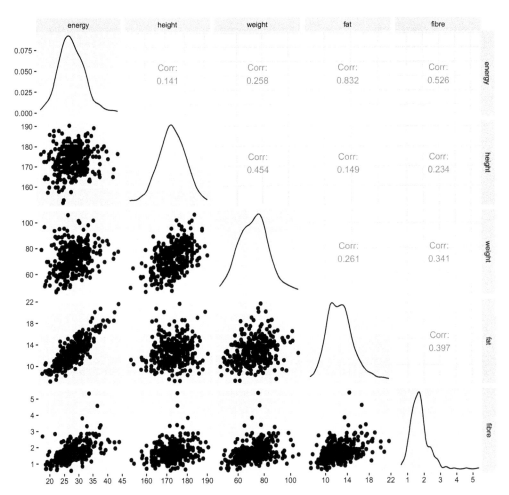

Figure 4.4 Scatter plot matrix of quantitative variables from the `diet` data. Note that fat and energy are the closest correlated variables, with an empirical correlation of 0.832.

It can be inspected by the `pairs` function from base R or the slightly more sophisticated `ggpairs`, which not only makes all pairwise scatter plots but also gives the marginal distributions and computes the correlations:

```
> library(ggplot2)
> library(GGally)
> ggpairs( diet, columns=9:13 )
```

> CODE EXPLAINED: We load the `ggplot2` and `GGally` packages; the latter requires the former. We then use the `ggpairs` function that makes all pairwise scatter plots of the variables indicated. We could also have used the indexing facilities for the columns of a data frame and used `ggpairs( diet[,9:13] )`.

If we put both `energy` and `fat` in the model (together with `height` which is by far the strongest predictor), we see that the standard errors of the coefficients are almost of the same magnitude as the the estimates themselves, so the effects of the two variables are 'non-significant':

```
> mc <- lm( weight ~ height + fat + energy, data = diet )
> round( cbind( ci.lin(mc)[,c(1:2,4)], cor( vcov(mc) ) ), 3 )
              Estimate StdErr     P (Intercept) height    fat energy
(Intercept)   -64.644 14.061 0.000        1.000 -1.000  0.824 -0.950
height          0.712  0.082 0.000       -1.000  1.000 -0.823  0.950
fat             0.450  0.397 0.257        0.824 -0.823  1.000 -0.958
energy          0.286  0.213 0.178       -0.950  0.950 -0.958  1.000
```

> CODE EXPLAINED: lm fits the model, and ci.lin extracts the parameters and the standard errors; here we also fish out the p-values (3rd column). Using cbind we put this next to the correlation matrix of the parameters; vcov extracts the variance–covariance matrix of the parameters, and cor converts it to a correlation matrix.

We see that the *estimates* of the effects of energy and fat are strongly *negatively* correlated, with a correlation of −0.958. This is because the *variables* are strongly *positively* correlated.

Loosely speaking, the variables energy and fat are strongly positively correlated and so have a strong common component. The corresponding two coefficients measure the joint effect of energy and fat, so if we were to increase the effect of energy a bit we would have to decrease the effect of fat accordingly, because of the common component. Hence the negative correlation between the estimates.

We saw that there were no 'significant' effects of either energy or fat, but this only means that there is little effect of energy as long as all other variables are in the model, including fat. And of course vice versa. But if we remove either of the variables, then the other one becomes strongly significant:

```
> round( ci.lin( update(mc,.~.-fat    ) ), 4 )
              Estimate   StdErr       z P     2.5%     97.5%
(Intercept) -65.5112  14.0464 -4.6639 0 -93.0417 -37.9807
height        0.7169   0.0814  8.8071 0   0.5574   0.8765
energy        0.4868   0.1181  4.1228 0   0.2554   0.7183
> round( ci.lin( update(mc,.~.-energy) ), 4 )
              Estimate   StdErr       z       P     2.5%     97.5%
(Intercept) -62.7741  14.0096 -4.4808 0e+00 -90.2324 -35.3157
height        0.7148   0.0816  8.7625 0e+00   0.5549   0.8747
fat           0.8947   0.2206  4.0553 1e-04   0.4623   1.3271
```

> CODE EXPLAINED: The function update fits a new model derived from an existing model; anything can be changed: response, explanatory variables, data, etc. Here we only change the explanatory variables in the model mc. The dots refer to the existing model, so the response variable and the explanatory variables are the same; in the first one fat is removed, while in the second energy is removed.
>
> In both cases we use ci.lin to extract parameters and coefficients.

The coefficients of energy and fat become larger in the models where only one of the variables is included. This is because one of the variables now has to carry the effect of both (via the correlation). At the same time the standard errors become smaller. These two phenomena are common when correlated variables are entered in a regression model.

They also illustrate the necessity to interpret effects estimated from multiple regression models always remembering that they are *conditional* on all the other effects in the model.

So there is no such thing as the effect of `fat`; it can only be interpreted conditional on the presence or absence of `energy` in the model.

A related phenomenon occur when a variable in a model is *perfectly* correlated with (a linear function of) other variables—that is, if there is a linear relationship. We can illustrate this by including the sum of `fat` and `energy` in the model:

```
> summary( update(mc,.~.+I(fat+energy)) )

Call:
lm(formula = weight ~ height + fat + energy + I(fat + energy),
    data = diet)

Residuals:
    Min      1Q  Median      3Q     Max
-21.072  -7.194  -0.183   6.505  26.534

Coefficients: (1 not defined because of singularities)
                Estimate Std. Error t value Pr(>|t|)
(Intercept)     -64.64396   14.06114  -4.597 6.12e-06
height            0.71153    0.08151   8.730  < 2e-16
fat               0.45019    0.39699   1.134    0.258
energy            0.28624    0.21265   1.346    0.179
I(fat + energy)        NA         NA      NA       NA

Residual standard error: 9.395 on 328 degrees of freedom
  (5 observations deleted due to missingness)
Multiple R-squared:  0.2482,    Adjusted R-squared:  0.2413
F-statistic:  36.1 on 3 and 328 DF,  p-value: < 2.2e-16
```

CODE EXPLAINED: We use the `update` function to add the sum of `fat` and `energy` as a new variable by using `I()`. `summary` is used to inspect the fitted model.

We see that the coefficients are unchanged, except for the variable we added where coefficient is NA. This is because the effect of this variable is already in the model, but it cannot be assigned a unique value. If we let β_e and β_f be the coefficients for `energy` and `fat` respectively, we have for any number δ

$$\beta_e\text{energy} + \beta_f\text{fat} = (\beta_e - \delta)\text{energy} + (\beta_f - \delta)\text{fat} + \delta(\text{energy} + \text{fat})$$

So we may claim that the coefficient (δ) to the sum of the two variables has any value we like, as long as we adjust the values for the effects of `energy` and `fat`.

We say that the parameter δ is *aliased*, meaning that it does not add anything to the model relative to the other parameters. It matters what order the variables are entered in the model; if we remove `fat` from the model and add it *after* the sum we see that it is now `fat` that is aliased:

```
> summary( update(mc, . ~ . -fat + I(fat+energy) + fat) )

Call:
lm(formula = weight ~ height + energy + I(fat + energy) + fat,
    data = diet)

Residuals:
    Min      1Q  Median      3Q     Max
-21.072  -7.194  -0.183   6.505  26.534
```

```
Coefficients: (1 not defined because of singularities)
                 Estimate Std. Error t value Pr(>|t|)
(Intercept)      -64.64396   14.06114  -4.597 6.12e-06
height             0.71153    0.08151   8.730  < 2e-16
energy            -0.16395    0.58589  -0.280   0.780
I(fat + energy)    0.45019    0.39699   1.134   0.258
fat                     NA         NA      NA      NA

Residual standard error: 9.395 on 328 degrees of freedom
  (5 observations deleted due to missingness)
Multiple R-squared:  0.2482,    Adjusted R-squared:  0.2413
F-statistic:  36.1 on 3 and 328 DF,  p-value: < 2.2e-16
```

Aliased coefficients occur when a variable (specifically, a column in the model matrix) is a linear function of the previous ones, previous meaning 'mentioned earlier in the model formula'. In the previous example we made `fat` have the role of being aliased.

Sometimes aliasing occurs because of a lack of data; there might be only one data point for a given job category, and so a model attempting to estimate a separate slope in each will be frustrated.

4.8 Logarithmic transformations

One of the most common transformations used, for both explanatory and response variables, is the logarithmic transformation, briefly the log-transform.

In order to explain how these work, we first explain the nature of the logarithmic functions.

4.8.1 *Logarithms*

There are many logarithm functions; they all have the property

$$\ell(y \times x) = \ell(y) + \ell(x), \qquad \ell(1) = 0$$

—the latter is really a consequence of the former; by setting $x = 1$ we get $\ell(y) = \ell(y \times 1) = \ell(y) + \ell(1)$, so $\ell(1)$ must be 0.

The *base* of a logarithm is the number b for which $\ell(b) = 1$; the logarithm with base b is normally denoted by $\log_b$, so $\log_b(b) = 1$. It is a mathematical fact that any two logarithm functions are proportional, so the logarithm with base b can be constructed from any other logarithm by

$$\log_b(x) = \log(x)/\log(b)$$

—which clearly has the desired property that if you replace x with b you get $\log_b(b) = 1$.

The *inverse* of the logarithm with base b is the *exponential* with base b, so

$$z = \log_b(y) \quad \Leftrightarrow \quad y = b^z$$

From a mathematical point of view this can be regarded as merely the definition of b^z.

The function `log` in R has an argument, `base`, which enables you to use any base you please. The logarithms with base 2 and base 10 are common, so they have their own functions, `log2`, respectively `log10`:

```
> x <- c(0.5,1,1.5,2,3,9:11)
> cbind( x, log=log(x), log2=log2(x),
+                     log10=log10(x),
+                     log1.5=log(x,base=1.5),
+                     log0.5=log(x,base=0.5) )
         x        log       log2      log10     log1.5     log0.5
[1,]   0.5 -0.6931472 -1.0000000 -0.3010300 -1.709511  1.0000000
[2,]   1.0  0.0000000  0.0000000  0.0000000  0.000000  0.0000000
[3,]   1.5  0.4054651  0.5849625  0.1760913  1.000000 -0.5849625
[4,]   2.0  0.6931472  1.0000000  0.3010300  1.709511 -1.0000000
[5,]   3.0  1.0986123  1.5849625  0.4771213  2.709511 -1.5849625
[6,]   9.0  2.1972246  3.1699250  0.9542425  5.419023 -3.1699250
[7,]  10.0  2.3025851  3.3219281  1.0000000  5.678874 -3.3219281
[8,]  11.0  2.3978953  3.4594316  1.0413927  5.913937 -3.4594316
```

CODE EXPLAINED: The x is filled with a set of illustrative values; cbind puts x side by side with columns of the logarithms of x. In order to get a readable output the columns are named. Note where the results are 1: at the base value of x. Also note that with a base less than 1 (here 0.5) we have a decreasing logarithm function.

The *natural* logarithm is defined by the property that its slope is 1 at $x = 1$. All logarithm functions go through (1,0) (because $\log(1) = 0$) but only one has slope 1 at this point. This property of the natural logarithm means that if h is small (in practical terms $|h| < 0.1$), then $\log(1 + h) \approx h$.

It turns out that this property implies that the base is e = 2.718282. The natural logarithm is normally denoted $\log(y)$; in R it is called log. Occasionally, $\log_e(y)$ or $\ln(y)$ is used to denote the natural logarithm. The inverse function is denoted $\exp(z)$ or e^z; in R it is called exp(z). If we want the base of the natural logarithm we just ask for exp(1), and if we want it really precisely, we can ask R to print in maximal precision (22 is the maximal allowed for digits here):

```
> options(digits=22)
> exp(1)

[1] 2.71828182845904509096

> options(digits=7)
> curve( log, from=0.2, to=4, lwd=3, xlim=c(0,4), xaxs="i" )
> abline( -1, 1 )
> abline( v=1, h=0 )
> abline( v=exp(1), h=1, lty="24" )
> axis( side=1, at=exp(1), labels="e" )
```

CODE EXPLAINED: options sets different parameters that determine how R behaves; the digits determines how many *significant* digits is printed. We reset the digits to the default of 7 in order to avoid messy output subsequently.

The function curve plots a given function (in this case the natural logarithm, log) over a given range of *x*es, here from 0.2 to 4, and lwd specifies the thickness of the line drawn. xlim gives the extent of the *x*-axis, and xaxs="i" specified that the axis is precisely from 0 to 4, without adding a bit in either end as is the default. This is to emphasize that the logarithm is only defined for $x > 0$, so it is meaningless to have an axis stretching below 0.

The first `abline` draws a straight line with intercept −1 and slope 1—the tangent of log(x) at 1; the second `abline` draws a vertical line at 1 and a horizontal line at 0, and the third `abline` draws dotted lines, horizontal at 1, and vertical at e. Finally the `axis` statement just puts a tick mark at exp(1) = e, and labels it 'e'.

4.8.2 Log transform of the response variable

One reason to transform the response variable with the logarithm may be that we want an interpretation of the covariate effects as multiplicative on the original scale. It might also be that the transform provided a better fit in a linear model. If we have a regression model for the log-transformed variable:

$$\log(y_i) = \alpha + \beta x_i + e_i$$

the interpretation is that an increase in x by 1 increases $\log(y)$ by β, or equivalently if we compare two persons, with a difference of 1 in x, the difference in the response will be

$$\beta = \log(y_1) - \log(y_0) = \log(y_1/y_0) \quad \Leftrightarrow \quad y_1/y_0 = \exp(\beta)$$

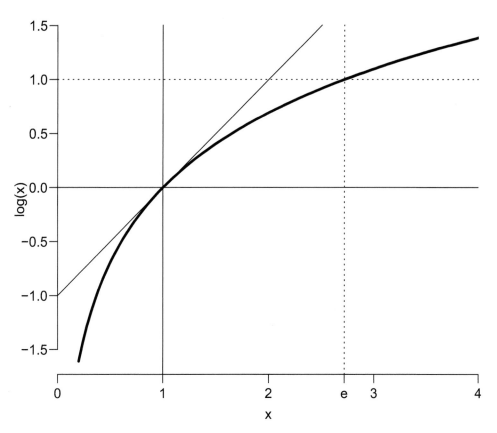

Figure 4.5 Graph of the natural logarithm. The line through (1,0) has slope 1, illustrating that the slope of the natural logarithm at 1 is 1. The dotted lines illustrate the base of the natural logarithm; it is 1 at e.

so in a model like this, $\exp(\beta)$ will represent the *relative* change in y for a unit change in x; the percentage change in y will be $(\exp(\beta) - 1) * 100$.

Suppose we want to see how weight changes in *relative* terms by height

```
> ml <- lm( log(weight) ~ height, data=diet )
> round( ci.lin( ml ), 4 )
            Estimate StdErr      z P   2.5%  97.5%
(Intercept)   2.3979 0.1999 11.9932 0 2.0061 2.7898
height        0.0108 0.0012  9.3860 0 0.0086 0.0131
> round( (ci.exp( ml, subset="height" )-1)*100, 1 )
       exp(Est.) 2.5% 97.5%
height       1.1  0.9   1.3
```

> CODE EXPLAINED: To get the percentage change in weight per cm height we use the natural log transform of weight as the response variable. The parameter β must then be transformed by $(\exp(\beta) - 1) \times 100$ to give the percentage change in weight per 1 cm in height. The `ci.exp` exponentiates the estimate and the confidence limits, so we subtract 1 and multiply by 100 to get the percentage weight change per centimeter height, with corresponding confidence intervals.

Here we see that the effect of 1 cm difference in height corresponds to a difference of 0.0108 in the natural log of weight. Translated to the relative scale this amounts to a weight change of 1.1% per cm of height, with quite a narrow confidence interval (0.9; 1.3)%/cm.

So log-transformation of the response variable gives *relative* effects on the response variable for absolute changes in the explanatory variable. Whether this is a sensible description is a subject-matter question, neither a mathematical nor a statistical one.

4.8.3 *Coefficient of variation*

Recall that one of the central assumptions in the general linear model is the single residual standard deviation; it is constant across the range of y. If we use the natural log of the response variable we are instead making an assumption that the $\log(y)$ has a constant standard deviation across the range of y.

A theorem from mathematical statistics states that if a variable z has mean μ_z and standard deviation σ_z, then $\log(z)$ has mean $\log(\mu_z)$ and standard deviation σ_z/μ_z, approximately at least.

Thus if we assume that the the standard deviation of $\log(y)$ is constant across the range of y, we assume that the ratio of the standard deviation to the mean of y, σ_y/μ_y, is constant across the range of y. In other words, the standard deviation of y, σ_y, is proportional to the mean of y, μ_y. The proportionality factor, which is the ratio of the standard deviation to the mean, is called the *coefficient of variation*, often abbreviated as CV:

$$CV = \sigma_y/\mu_y \quad \Leftrightarrow \quad \sigma_y = CV\,\mu_y$$

Under the assumption that the standard deviation of the weight is proportional to the mean weight, an estimate of the proportionality factor will be the residual standard deviation from the model for the log-weight. This is found as the component `sigma` in the list that is returned by `summary(ml)`:

```
> summary(ml)$sigma
[1] 0.1344238
```

Here we see that the residual standard error is 0.13; this is the coefficient of variation, so under the assumptions of the model, the standard deviation of the weight is about 13% of the mean weight, across the range of weight.

Occasionally, the coefficient of variation is seen computed as the empirical standard deviation divided by the empirical mean:

```
> with( subset( diet, !is.na(weight) ), sd(weight)/mean(weight) )
[1] 0.1485824
```

We see that this is not far off the value of the (residual) standard deviation from the model for the log-weight, and actually neither is far from the standard deviation of the log-weight overall:

```
> sd( log(diet$weight), na.rm=TRUE )
[1] 0.15095
```

The two latter calculations are just relating the overall s.d. to the overall mean and so are based on an assumption that the mean is the same in the entire sample, so the proportionality interpretation is a bit moot.

The first CV we computed is from the model m1 where the mean actually varies and therefore has an interpretation as a proportionality factor linking a varying standard deviation to a varying mean weight.

The reason that the difference between the simple and the model-based CV is small is that the model explains very little of the variation in weight. If the range of weight had been larger and height more predictive the difference would have been larger.

4.8.4 *Log transform of an explanatory variable*

In some circumstances it will be relevant to log-transform the explanatory variable(s). It may be because the model will fit better or because the distribution of an explanatory variable is very right-skewed so a relative effect of the variable appears more credible. This is an empirical question, and no general guidelines can be given as to when to log-transform an explanatory variable.

As mentioned previously, in regression models there are no distributional assumptions for the explanatory variables—the models are for the *conditional* distribution of the response *given* the values of the explanatory variables. So the reason to log-transform an explanatory variable is never to obtain a particular distributional form, but rather to obtain a description of the effect that is clinically relevant.

If we transform by the base b logarithm we will have a parameter estimate that corresponds to the change in y for a change of 1 in $\log_b(x)$. If we compare two persons with difference of 1 in log_b-transformed values of x we see that:

$$1 = \log_b(x_1) - \log_b(x_0) = \log_b(x_1/x_0) \quad \Leftrightarrow \quad x_1/x_0 = b$$

because b is the base of the logarithm. So we will get the interpretation as the effect of a b-fold increase in x if we transform x by the logarithm with base b. This is why we do not normally use the natural log for transforming explanatory variables. We would use the log to base 2 or 10, depending on whether a relevant range in the explanatory variable were 2-fold or 10-fold.

If we use the height–weight example, a 2-fold difference in height is presumably not a relevant effect to report; even a 10% difference in weight is quite large. If we want to report the effect of a 10% height increase on weight, we must use the logarithm with base 1.1:

```
> me <- lm( weight ~ log(height,base=1.1), data=diet )
> round( ci.lin( me ), 4 )
                        Estimate  StdErr      z P      2.5%      97.5%
(Intercept)           -607.9914 73.3948 -8.2838 0 -751.8426 -464.1401
log(height, base = 1.1)  12.5836  1.3570  9.2728 0    9.9238   15.2433
```

The interpretation of the coefficient to the log variable here is that weight increases by 12 kg for a 10% increase in height. So transforming explanatory variables will produce absolute effects of the response variable for a relative change of the explanatory variable. The size of the relative change reflected in the parameter estimate is determined by the base of the logarithm used.

In generalized linear models such as logistic regression or Poisson models, transforming an explanatory variable is perfectly sensible; interpretation will be the same—the effect of a relative change in the explanatory variable.

4.8.5 *Log transform of both the response and explanatory variables*

Of course it is possible to transform both the response and explanatory variables; just remember that the response variable must be transformed by the natural log, and the explanatory variable by a logarithm with a base that represents a subject-matter relevant change in the explanatory variable—for the height we use the base 1.1:

```
> mb <- lm( log(weight) ~ log(height,base=1.1), data=diet )
> round( (ci.exp( mb, subset="height" )-1)*100, 4 )
                        exp(Est.)    2.5%    97.5%
log(height, base = 1.1)    19.522 15.1649  24.0441
```

Thus we see that a 10% increase in height is associated with a 19.5% increase in weight.

CHAPTER 5

Analysis of follow-up data

The mortality rate data we looked at in section 2.2 (p. 42) were *aggregated* from data on a large number of individuals, all of whom contribute some risk time (that adds up to the 300,000 person-years), and some of whom contribute the 2,648 deaths. Here we explain how this type of data comes about from the individuals in a cohort followed over time.

At the same time we explain the likelihood from a follow-up study and why we can analyse rates using Poisson regression.

5.1 Basic data structure

Follow-up refers to the process of monitoring persons over time for occurrence of a (set of) prespecified event(s). The simplest example is following persons for the occurrence of death. Practical data collection is often via look-up in registers or databases.

The basic requirements for recordings in a follow-up study is

- Date of entry to the study—the first date a person is known to be alive and at risk of having an event.
- Date of exit from the study—the last date a person is known to be alive and at risk of having an event.
- The status of the person at the exit date—with or without event.

It is assumed that the event terminates the follow-up, so we are implicitly referring to events like death or diagnosis of a chronic disease, where a person ceases to be at risk of the event if it occurs.

In the Epi package is the dataset DMlate:

```
> library( Epi )
> library( popEpi )
> data( DMlate )
> str( DMlate )
'data.frame':   10000 obs. of  7 variables:
 $ sex  : Factor w/ 2 levels "M","F": 2 1 2 2 1 2 1 1 2 1 ...
 $ dobth: num  1940 1939 1918 1965 1933 ...
 $ dodm : num  1999 2003 2005 2009 2009 ...
 $ dodth: num  NA NA NA NA NA ...
 $ dooad: num  NA 2007 NA NA NA ...
 $ doins: num  NA NA NA NA NA NA NA NA NA NA ...
 $ dox  : num  2010 2010 2010 2010 2010 ...
```

This dataset represents follow-up of a random sample of 10,000 diabetes patients in Denmark diagnosed after 1995, followed till the end of 2009. Random noise has been

Epidemiology with R. Bendix Carstensen, Oxford University Press (2021). © Bendix Carstensen.
DOI: 10.1093/oso/9780198841326.003.0006

added to all dates in order to make persons untraceable. A brief overview of the data can be seen from the first few lines of data—each line represents the follow-up of one person:

```
> head( DMlate )
        sex     dobth     dodm     dodth    dooad doins        dox
50185     F 1940.256 1998.917       NA       NA    NA 2009.997
307563    M 1939.218 2003.309       NA 2007.446    NA 2009.997
294104    F 1918.301 2004.552       NA       NA    NA 2009.997
336439    F 1965.225 2009.261       NA       NA    NA 2009.997
245651    M 1932.877 2008.653       NA       NA    NA 2009.997
216824    F 1927.870 2007.886 2009.923       NA    NA 2009.923
```

The overall number of deaths, follow-up time, and mortality rates by sex can be shown using stat.table:

```
> stat.table( index = sex,
+          contents = list( D = sum( !is.na(dodth) ),
+                           Y = sum( dox-dodm ),
+                        rate = ratio(!is.na(dodth), dox-dodm, 1000) ),
+             margin = TRUE,
+               data = DMlate )

 ----------------------------------
 sex           D        Y     rate
 ----------------------------------
 M       1345.00 27614.21    48.71
 F       1158.00 26659.05    43.44


 Total   2503.00 54273.27    46.12
 ----------------------------------
```

> CODE EXPLAINED: The index argument defines the cells of the table, in this case three; one for each sex, plus 1 because we asked for a margin (margin=TRUE). The contents argument defines what goes in each cell of the table, in this case three numbers labelled D, Y, and rate. The expression !is.na(dodth) is a logical indicator of whether the date of death (dodth) is non-missing. This is converted from FALSE/TRUE to 0/1 when summed, giving the total number of deaths. dox-dodm is simply the follow-up time for each person (in years), so we have the number of deaths and the person-years, and finally the ratio of the two multiplied by 1000, the latter giving the mortality rate per 1000 PY.

The overall mortality rate is 46.1 deaths per 1000 person-years. In making this calculation we already implicitly imposed a statistical model describing the data, namely, the model which assumes a constant mortality rate for all persons during the study period. The single entries are from a model that assumes that mortality rates only differ by sex. While this model is clearly wrong for almost any purpose, it serves as an essential building block in derivation of more realistic models.

5.2 Probability model

A (theoretical) mortality *rate* is the probability of death in a small interval, *relative* to the length of the interval, usually denoted by λ (the Greek letter lambda):

$$\lambda = \mathrm{P}\{\text{death in } (t, t + \mathrm{d}t] \,|\, \text{alive at } t\} / \mathrm{d}t$$

If we assume λ is known, for example $\lambda = 46.1/1000$ years, i.e. an assumption that the mortality rate does not depend on t (persons' age or calendar time at follow-up), we could generate a follow-up dataset by simulation:

1. Start with all the persons entering the study.
2. The first day of follow-up each person has a probability of dying which is $\lambda \times 1\text{day} = 46.1/1000\text{y} \times 1\text{day}$ which is equal to $46.1 \times (1/365250) = 0.0001262$—taking leap years into account, there are 365.25 days in a year and hence 365,250 days in 1,000 years.[1]
3. For each person, simulate a 0/1 variable with probability of 1 (=death) being 0.000126. If this is turns out to be 1 the person is considered dead this day and removed from further calculation.
4. The survivors are subjected to the same procedure next day, etc.

Thus after, say, 15×365 days, we have generated a *simulated* survival study where a certain number of persons have been followed for 15 years subject to a constant mortality rate of 46.1 per 1000 years.

This is one way of describing a probability model as a machinery that prescribes how to simulate a dataset with given theoretical quantities (such as a rate) as input.

5.2.1 Data

In practical data analysis we go the other way round and compute the *probability* of seeing the data we actually observed, assuming we know the probability model that generated the data. This probability is what we introduced as the *likelihood* in Chapter 3.

The likelihood for a follow-up study depends on the size of the mortality rate, and we choose the value of the mortality parameter that assigns the highest probability to our observed data, the *maximum likelihood* estimate. In this sense, the mortality rate is the *parameter* in the model, the quantity we want to *estimate*.

The probability of seeing the amount of follow-up time and number of deaths in the entire study is the *product* of the probabilities of seeing the follow-up for each person, because persons are assumed independent.

5.2.2 Likelihood for a rate

Thus it remains to compute the probability of the observation from a single person. Suppose a person is alive from t_e (entry) to t_x (exit) and that the person's status at t_x is d, where $d = 0$ means alive and $d = 1$ means dead. If we choose three time-points, t_1, t_2, t_3 between t_e and t_x, standard use of conditional probability (formally, repeated use of Bayes' formula) gives

$$
\begin{aligned}
\mathrm{P}\{d \text{ at } t_x \,|\, \text{entry at } t_e\} = \; & \mathrm{P}\{\text{survive } (t_e, t_1] \,|\, \text{alive at } t_e\} \\
& \times \mathrm{P}\{\text{survive } (t_1, t_2] \,|\, \text{alive at } t_1\} \\
& \times \mathrm{P}\{\text{survive } (t_2, t_3] \,|\, \text{alive at } t_2\} \\
& \times \mathrm{P}\{d \text{ at } t_x \,|\, \text{alive at } t_3\}
\end{aligned}
$$

---

[1] Actually, there are only 97 leap years every 400 years, so in 1,000 calendar-years there are 365,242.5 days. But we are dealing with contemporary *person*-years, and in the period 1901–2099 every 4th year is a leap year (1900 and 2100 are not leap years, but 2000 is), so in practical terms we are dealing with a period where there are 365.25 days on average per year.

By choosing more intermediate time-points we can make the intervals arbitrarily small, so we just need to derive the probability of surviving a small piece of time, as a function of the mortality rate λ. From the definition of a rate we have (conditional on being alive at t)

$$P\{\text{death during } (t, t+h]\} \approx \lambda h$$
$$\Rightarrow P\{\text{survive } (t, t+h]\} \approx 1 - \lambda h$$

where the approximation gets better the smaller the interval is. Suppose we have survival for a time span $y = t_x - t_e$ and that this is subdivided in N intervals, each of length $h = y/N$; then the survival probability for the entire span from t_e to t_x is the product of probabilities of surviving each of the small intervals:

$$P\{\text{survive } t_e \text{ to } t_x\} \approx (1 - \lambda h)^N$$

If λh is small (and it will be if h is sufficiently small), then, using the mathematical approximation $1 - \lambda h \approx \exp(-\lambda h)$, we get

$$P\{\text{survive } t_e \text{ to } t_x\} \approx \exp(-\lambda h N) = \exp(-\lambda y), \tag{5.1}$$

so the contribution to the likelihood from a person observed for a time span of length y is $\exp(-\lambda y)$, and the contribution to the log-likelihood from each interval is therefore $-\lambda y$.

If we observe a person dying, the contribution to the likelihood from the last interval will be the probability of dying in the interval, which is λh and the log-likelihood contribution from the last interval for this person is then $\log(\lambda h) = \log(\lambda) + \log(h)$.

The total likelihood for one person is the product of all these terms from the follow-up intervals for one person; and the log-likelihood (ℓ) is the sum of them, in total,

$$\ell(\lambda) = -\lambda \sum_i y_i + \sum_i d_i \log(\lambda) + \sum_i d_i \log(y_i)$$

where y_i is observation time (risk time or person-years) and d_i the death indicator (0/1) for the ith interval. We are out to estimate λ, so terms that does not involve λ can be ignored—such as the last term. Thus we have established that the contribution to the log-likelihood from a single person's follow-up is the sum of a number of terms of the form $d \log(\lambda) - \lambda y$, where d is the event indicator (0/1) and y the length of a small interval.

Now, the log-likelihood contribution from a Poissonvariate d with mean λh is $d \log(\lambda h) - \lambda h$, which is the same as the likelihood for d events during h follow-up time with rate λ (except for the term $d \log(h)$ that does not depend on the parameter λ). This means that maximum-likelihood estimation can be done using the estimation function $\texttt{glm}$ if we pretend that the ds are independent Poisson variates with means λy.

Note that the only feature we use is that the likelihood is a *product* of terms; there is no assumption about the contributions being independent. It is the product that makes the likelihood for a constant rate over many small intervals *look like* the likelihood for many independent Poisson variates (the d_is). But there is not a one-to-one correspondence between likelihoods and models; here we have two different models that have the same likelihood. And in practical estimation we only use the likelihood, not the model.

5.2.3 *Estimates of rates and rate ratios*

In the case where the rate is assumed constant, the Poisson likelihood leads to the estimate

$$\hat{\lambda} = D/Y, \qquad \text{s.e.}\left(\log(\hat{\lambda})\right) = 1/\sqrt{D}$$

so that approximate 95% confidence intervals for the log-rate and the rate are

$$\log(D/Y) \pm 2 \times (1/\sqrt{D}) \qquad \Leftrightarrow \qquad D/Y \stackrel{\times}{\div} \exp\left(2 \times (1/\sqrt{D})\right) \qquad (5.2)$$

If we have two rates based on D_1, Y_1 and D_0, Y_0 (events, person-time) and the two bodies of data are independent, then the log-rate-ratio is the difference of the log-rates, and hence the *variance* of the log-rate-ratio is $1/D_0 + 1/D_1$, and by that token a 95% c.i. for the rate ratio is

$$(D_1/Y_1) / (D_0/Y_0) \stackrel{\times}{\div} \exp\left(2(1/D_1 + 1/D_0)\right) \qquad (5.3)$$

The terms $\exp\left(2 \times (1/\sqrt{D})\right)$ and $\exp\left(2(1/D_1 + 1/D_0)\right)$ are occasionally termed 'error factor'. Simple applications of these formulae are on pp. 120 and 122.

5.3 Representation of follow-up data

This representation of the *likelihood* of the follow-up of a person over several small intervals is what we shall use in the `Lexis` objects used for representation of the follow-up *data*.

In the `Epi` package, follow-up data are represented in a data frame by adding some extra variables to it. The extra variables are used for keeping track of what state persons are in (alive or dead) and what time it is. Such a data frame is called a `Lexis` object [9].[2] This special structure of a `Lexis` object is used to make handling of the follow-up information easier.

Follow-up data basically consist of a time of entry, a time of exit, and an indication of the status at exit (normally either 'Alive' or 'Dead'). Implicitly is also assumed as a status *during* the follow-up (usually 'Alive').

Note that time comes in two guises: one is the *risk* time (in demography 'exposure'), and the other is the time-*scale*. The risk time is '*how long* have you been alive' (exposed to potential death); the time-scale is '*when* were you alive', meaning for example age or calendar time. The risk time is part of the outcome measurement (it is the denominator of the rate), whereas the time-scale is an explanatory variable. We will usually be interested in how rates vary along some time-scale, age, or calendar time, for example, so in most analyses we will be using both risk time and time-scales.

5.3.1 *Lexis object for follow-up data*

As an example we use the `DMlate` data from the `Epi` package; it is a dataset of 10,000 randomly selected patients from the Danish Diabetes register diagnosed after 1995, but where all dates have been randomly perturbed so no persons are identifiable. For the `DMlate` data we can construct a `Lexis` object with age as time-scale by

```
> data( DMlate )
> Ldm <- Lexis( entry = list( age=dodm-dobth ),
+                exit = list( age=dox-dobth ),
+         exit.status = factor( !is.na(dodth), labels=c("Alive","Dead") ),
+                data = DMlate )
NOTE: entry.status has been set to "Alive" for all.
NOTE: Dropping  4  rows with duration of follow up < tol
```

---

[2] Named after the German demographer Wilhelm Lexis (1837–1914), who in his book *Einleitung in die Theorie der Bevölkerungsstatistik* devised what is usually called the Lexis diagram for graphical representation of follow-up on several times-cales.

```
> summary( Ldm )
Transitions:
     To
From    Alive Dead  Records:   Events: Risk time:   Persons:
  Alive  7497 2499      9996      2499   54273.27       9996
```

> CODE EXPLAINED: The `entry` argument is a *named* list which defines the name of the time-scale (`age`) and the entry point of each person measured on this time-scale (`dodm-dobth`, age at date of diagnosis). The `exit` argument gives the exit time on the time-scale (`dox-dobth`, age at exit); the name of the element in this list must match the one in the `entry` list. The status at the end of follow-up is given by the `exit.status` argument; here `!is.na(dodth)` is a logical variable, where FALSE<TRUE so FALSE is coded 'Alive' and TRUE coded 'Dead'. There are 4 persons who have `dodm=dox`, and thus 0 follow-up time; these 4 are excluded and hence only 9996 persons are left.
>
> The `summary` provides an overview of transitions from `Alive` to `Dead`, risk time, and the number of persons in the study. Risk time is measured in the units in which the `age` (the time-scale) was entered, in this case years.

The `Lexis` machinery also accommodates multiple time-scales; if we want to add calendar time we would do the following:

```
> Ldm <- Lexis( entry = list( age=dodm-dobth,
+                              per=dodm ),
+               exit = list( per=dox ),
+        exit.status = factor( !is.na(dodth), labels=c("Alive","Dead") ),
+               data = DMlate )
NOTE: entry.status has been set to "Alive" for all.
NOTE: Dropping  4  rows with duration of follow up < tol
> summary( Ldm, t=T )
Transitions:
     To
From    Alive Dead  Records:   Events: Risk time:   Persons:
  Alive  7497 2499      9996      2499   54273.27       9996

Timescales:
age per
 " "   " "
```

> CODE EXPLAINED: The `entry` argument can be a *named* list with the entry points on the different times-cales we want to use (`age`, age and `per`, calendar time). It defines the name of the time-scales and the entry points on these. The `exit` argument gives the exit time on *one* of the time-scales, so the name of the element in this list must match one of those in the `entry` list. This is sufficient, because the follow-up time on all time-scales is the same, in this case `dox-dodm`. The summary would be the same as time-scales are ignored in the summary, but adding `t=T` (shorthand for `timeScales=TRUE`) lists the names of the defined time-scales.

Now take a look at the resulting data frame:

```
> oo <- options(digits=5)
> head( Ldm )[,1:9]
           age     per lex.dur lex.Cst lex.Xst lex.id sex  dobth    dodm
50185   58.661 1998.9 11.08008   Alive   Alive      1   F 1940.3 1998.9
307563  64.090 2003.3  6.68857   Alive   Alive      2   M 1939.2 2003.3
294104  86.251 2004.6  5.44559   Alive   Alive      3   F 1918.3 2004.6
336439  44.036 2009.3  0.73648   Alive   Alive      4   F 1965.2 2009.3
245651  75.775 2008.7  1.34428   Alive   Alive      5   M 1932.9 2008.7
216824  80.016 2007.9  2.03696   Alive    Dead      6   F 1927.9 2007.9
> options( oo )
```

CODE EXPLAINED: The options is merely used to make the output a bit more compact. If we assign options to an object, here oo, this can be used to restore the options to the previous state later. head just shows the first 6 records and [,1:9] selects columns 1 through 9. Note that Lexis created the two time-scale variables age and per as well as the risk time in lex.dur (duration), lex.Cst (Current state) the state where the risk time is spent, lex.Xst (eXit state) the state to which the persons moves after the lex.dur time in lex.Cst, and lex.id, an id variable for book keeping.

It is possible to get a visualization of the follow-up along the time-scales chosen by using the plot method for Lexis objects. Ldm is an object of *class* Lexis, so using the function plot() on it means that R will look for the function plot.Lexis and use this function:

```
> plot( Ldm )
```

CODE EXPLAINED: The plot really invokes plot.Lexis, since Ldm is an object of class Lexis. It will produce a Lexis diagram, where each record is represented by a line segment starting at the point of the value of the two first time-scales, and stretching lex.dur to the end on both time-scales. For example, for the person with lex.id=1 the segment will be from $(58.66, 1998.9)$ to $(58.66 + 11.08, 1998.9 + 11.08)$.

Since age is the first of the time-scales this is used as the *x*-axis, and the second per as the *y*-axis, as seen in the left panel of Figure 5.1, which may not be what you want.

Scaling of Lexis diagrams

The following is a bit esoteric, and can be skipped if you are not desperately interested in slick Lexis diagrams. The function plot.Lexis allows quite a bit of control over the output, and a points.Lexis function makes it possible to plot the end-points of follow-up:

```
> ypi <- 11 # years per inch
> pdf( "./graph/fudat-Ldm-xtra.pdf", width=25/ypi+1, height=100/ypi+1 )
> par( mai=c(3,3,1,1)/4, mgp=c(3,1,0)/1.6 )
> plot( Ldm, 2:1, lwd=1,
+       grid=list(1990+0:5*5,1:19*5), lty.grid=1, col.grid=gray(0.7),
+       xlim=c(1990,2015), xaxs="i",
+       ylim=c(   0, 100), yaxs="i", las=1 )
> points( Ldm, 2:1, pch=c(NA,16)[Ldm$lex.Xst], col="black", cex=0.6 )
> dev.off()
null device
          1
```

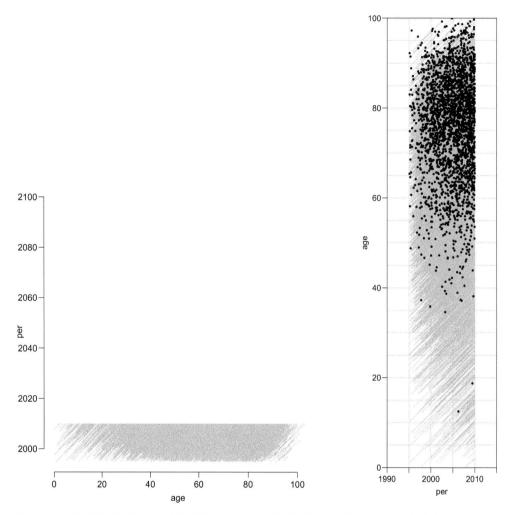

Figure 5.1 (Left) Default Lexis plot of the diabetes data. (Right panel:) Customized plot of the same data, adjusting the physical size of time-scales to be identical.

CODE EXPLAINED: The `mai` argument to `par()` gives the `margin` in `inches` (in order bottom, left, top, right), so the sum of the right and left margins is 1 inch ((3 + 1)/4), as is the sum of the top and bottom margins. Therefore when we in the `plot` specify axes to have an extent of 25, respectively 100 years, we can use the `width` and `height` arguments to the graphics driver `pdf` to specify the total size so that 11 years has an extent of 1 inch in both directions (the variable `ypi`, years per inch)—the +1 taking care of the margins.

The arguments `xaxs` and `yaxs` in `plot` are set to `"i"` assures the axes have the exact extent required (normally a little extra is added). The second argument gives the ordering of time-scales; in `Ldm`, age is the first and calendar time the second, but we want the second to be on the *x*-axis and the first to be on the *y*-axis.

The `grid` argument creates the grid behind the life lines. The `points` function *adds* points at the *end* of the life lines, ordering of the time-scales as for `plot`. `lex.Xst` is a factor with levels `Alive` and `Dead`, and in R indexing with a factor is the same as using the *number* of the factor levels as index, so persons `Alive` at the end of follow-up will be plotted with symbol type NA (none that is) and those who are Dead at the end will be have a point of type 16, which is a filled dot. cex regulates the size of the plotting symbol.

5.4 Splitting the follow-up time along a time-scale

As we saw in the derivation of the likelihood for follow-up data, the likelihood contribution from a single person's follow-up can be subdivided in contributions from sub-intervals of the follow-up. The point being that this allows us to use a separate rate parameter for each interval; in this case we will subdivide data into small intervals by age.

This can be achieved by either the splitLexis from the Epi package (note that the function is *not* called split.Lexis) or splitMulti from the popEpi package. This requires that the time-scale and the breakpoints on this time-scale be supplied:

```
> library( popEpi )
> Xdm <- splitLexis( Ldm, "age", breaks=0:100 )
> Mdm <- splitMulti( Ldm, age=0:100, )
> summary( Ldm )
Transitions:
     To
From    Alive Dead  Records:  Events: Risk time:  Persons:
  Alive 7497 2499      9996     2499   54273.27       9996
> summary( Xdm )
Transitions:
     To
From    Alive Dead  Records:  Events: Risk time:  Persons:
  Alive 61622 2499     64121    2499   54273.27       9996
> summary( Mdm )
Transitions:
     To
From    Alive Dead  Records:  Events: Risk time:  Persons:
  Alive 61620 2495     64115    2495   54266.14       9995
> subset( Ldm, lex.id==151 )[,1:6]
            age       per lex.dur lex.Cst lex.Xst lex.id
217034 60.1807 1999.051 3.017112   Alive    Dead    151
> subset( Mdm, lex.id==151 )[,1:6]
   lex.id      age       per   lex.dur lex.Cst lex.Xst
1:    151 60.1807 1999.051 0.8193018   Alive   Alive
2:    151 61.0000 1999.871 1.0000000   Alive   Alive
3:    151 62.0000 2000.871 1.0000000   Alive   Alive
4:    151 63.0000 2001.871 0.1978097   Alive    Dead
```

CODE EXPLAINED: splitLexis requires that we specify which time-scale we want to split along (in this case age), and the points on the time-scale where we want follow-up split (breaks=). The splitMulti from the popEpi package does the same with a more elegant syntax; for large datasets it is also (much) faster, it returns a data.table and not a data.frame, but the difference is slight.

By default splitMulti chops off follow-up time outside the range of the supplied breaks, which may or may not be what you want, see ?splitMulti. splitLexis has no such facility; it always keeps all the risk time. Hence, in this case we observe that the total risk time is slightly smaller in the Mdm object coming from splitMulti.

The subset takes the subsets of the Lexis objects that concern person 151, and prints these, albeit only the first six variables.

We see from the summarys that the number of persons, the amount of risk time, and the number of dead are the same in the original dataset and in the split one (well, almost, due to the chopping behaviour of splitMulti), but the number of records is much larger in the split data. From the listing of persons with lex.id 151, we see that the person's follow-up is subdivided at exact ages 61, 62, and 63, that the follow-up is divided over the 4 intervals, and finally that the three first intervals have an exit status Alive (in lex.Xst) whereas only the last interval has exit status Dead.

The resulting dataset is much larger than the previous one, but represents the same amount of risk time and the same number of deaths. We can tabulate the dataset by sex and age:

```
> astab <- xtabs( cbind( D = (lex.Xst=="Dead"),
+                        Y = lex.dur )
+                 ~ sex + floor(age),
+                 data = Mdm )
> str( astab )
 'xtabs' num [1:2, 1:100, 1:2] 0 0 0 0 0 0 0 0 0 0 ...
 - attr(*, "dimnames")=List of 3
  ..$ sex       : chr [1:2] "M" "F"
  ..$ floor(age): chr [1:100] "0" "1" "2" "3" ...
  ..$           : chr [1:2] "D" "Y"
 - attr(*, "call")= language xtabs(formula = cbind(D = (lex.Xst == "Dead"),
   Y = lex.dur) ~ sex + floor(age), data = Mdm)
> round( ftable( astab[,51:55,], row.vars=2 ),1 )
            sex     M              F
                    D     Y        D     Y
floor(age)
50                  5.0 453.3    0.0 337.5
51                  6.0 471.7    2.0 357.1
52                  7.0 508.5    6.0 385.8
53                  9.0 559.3    3.0 413.7
54                  5.0 608.2    8.0 438.1
```

CODE EXPLAINED: xtabs makes a table classified by the variables on the r.h.s. of the tilde ('~'), the entries are the *sum* of each of the columns on the l.h.s., in this case the deaths (D) defined as counts of records with lex.Xst equal to 'Dead' and the sum of the person-years (Y) from the variable lex.dur.

str shows that the result is a 3-dimensional structure: a table classified by age, sex, and the left-hand side of the formula (D resp. Y).

ftable (shorthand for flat table) prints the part of the table for ages 50–54, with the age-dimension as rows and the other two other dimensions as columns.

We could have achieved this by stat.table too; the difference is that stat.table only allows 2 dimensions, whereas xtabs allows any number; on the other hand, xtabs only does the sum of the variables, whereas stat.table also accommodates other summaries.

We can use this aggregated data to estimate the age-specific rates for men and women separately:

```
> a1 <- 0:99 # the 1-year age-classes
> mold <- glm( astab["M",,"D"] ~ factor(a1) - 1,
+              offset = log(astab["M",,"Y"]),
+              family = poisson )
> str( astab["M",,] )
 'table' num [1:100, 1:2] 0 0 0 0 0 0 0 0 0 0 ...
 - attr(*, "dimnames")=List of 2
  ..$ floor(age): chr [1:100] "0" "1" "2" "3" ...
  ..$           : chr [1:2] "D" "Y"
> mm <- glm( astab["M",,] ~ factor(a1) - 1, family = poisreg )
> mf <- glm( astab["F",,] ~ factor(a1) - 1, family = poisreg )
```

> CODE EXPLAINED: The fitting used to create `mold` is the 'classical' way of fitting a Poisson model to rates, using the number of events (deaths, D) as outcome, in this case `astab["M",,"D"]`, and the log of the person-years in `astab["M",,"Y"]` as offset, both of which are numerical vectors of length 100. The r.h.s. of the model formula specifies that we want one coefficient per age class (`a1`); the `-1` indicating that there should be no intercept in the model so that all parameters are log-rates, one per age class.
>
> The `poisreg` family used to fit the model `mm` has a simpler and more intuitive syntax; the outcome variable (the l.h.s. of the formula) must be a two-column matrix with event count as the first and risk time as the second, precisely what `astab["M",,]` is. You can check the syntax using `?poisreg`.

In some systems we get a warning of either 'algorithm did not converge' or 'fitted values of 0 occurred'; this is because some of the age classes have 0 counts, and the estimated rates there should be 0, which on the log-scale is $-\infty$. What happens is that the `glm` tries to accommodate this, but only until estimated rates get sufficiently close to 0 ($\exp(-27) \approx 1.4 \times 10^{-12}$). We can see that the two different ways of fitting the model behave slightly differently, but also that the estimates of log-rates actually are the log of empirical rates:

```
> cbind( poisson = coef(mold),
+        poisreg = coef(mm),
+               astab["M",,],
+        empirical = log(astab["M",,"D"]/astab["M",,"Y"]) )[35:38,]
              poisson    poisreg  D       Y   empirical
factor(a1)34  -4.732487  -4.732487 1 113.5777  -4.732487
factor(a1)35 -31.081271 -27.302585 0 118.9480       -Inf
factor(a1)36 -31.190549 -27.302585 0 132.6831       -Inf
factor(a1)37  -3.941083  -3.941083 3 154.4230  -3.941083
```

> CODE EXPLAINED: `cbind` puts columns next to each other; when we precede the specification of a column with a name this will be used for annotation of the column. The two first columns are the estimates from the Poisson models using the two different families `poisson` and `poisreg`. At first glance they look different, but the numbers $-31.xx$ and $-27.xx$ are just approximations to $\log(0) = -\infty$; the rates are 0, and so the log-rates are $-\infty$. The indexing `[35:38,]` at the end just selects rows from 35 to 38—rows are indicated before the comma, columns after, omission means 'all'.

5.5 Smooth age-effects for rates

With the fitted model we get very little new beyond the empirical mortality rates except that it is a handy way of computing confidence intervals for the empirical rates. However, many of the empirical rates are 0, so these are hardly relevant; we do not really believe that the mortality is exactly 0 just because no deaths were observed. What is relevant is to devise a *model* for for the mortality rates as a function of age.

This is done in a similar way to the modelling of the age-specific prevalence of diabetes in Chapter 3.

```
> A <- 0:99+0.5 # midpoints of age-classes
> sm <- glm( astab["M",,] ~ Ns( A, knots=c(20,40,60,70,80,90) ),
+            family=poisreg )
> sf <- glm( astab["F",,] ~ Ns( A, knots=c(20,40,60,70,80,90) ),
+            family=poisreg )
```

> CODE EXPLAINED: The Ns produces a *natural spline*; a function which is a 3rd degree polynomial between the knots, and a linear function before the first and after the last knot, and which is constrained to be nicely smooth *at* the knots. A more detailed explanation of splines is found in section 6.4.4, p. 130.

Once we have fitted models for mortality for men and women, we can extract the fitted values (the rates) and plot them together:

```
> nd <- data.frame( A=seq(10,99,0.5) )
> pm <- ci.pred( sm, nd )
> pf <- ci.pred( sf, nd )
> matshade( nd$A, cbind( pm, pf )*1000, plot=TRUE,
+           col=c("blue","red"), lwd=2,
+           log="y", ylim=c(0.5,300), las=1,
+           xlab="Age", ylab="DM mortality per 1000 PY" )
```

> CODE EXPLAINED: nd is a data frame with the variables in the model—in this case only one, A, the age. ci.pred provides predictions with confidence intervals from the model (as rates per 1 year); the result has as many rows as the nd data frame, so pm and pf hold the predicted mortality rates for men resp. women in ages 10, 10.5, 11, etc. matshade plots the age (nd$A) on the *x*-axis and the predicted rates (scaled to per 1000 person-years) on the *y*-axis with a 95% confidence interval as a shaded area around the curve. The other parameters to matshade have the same effects as used in plot or par.

5.5.1 *Disaggregated data*

The data we analysed were tabulated (using xtabs) from the dataset where we subdivided the follow-up data in one-year intervals. But we might as well have fitted the model using the original (disaggregated) data, that is Mdm:

```
> summary( Mdm, t=T )

Transitions:
      To
From    Alive Dead  Records:  Events: Risk time:  Persons:
  Alive 61620 2495     64115     2495   54266.14      9995
```

```
Timescales:
age per
 " "   " "
> xm <- glm( cbind(lex.Xst=="Dead",lex.dur)
+               ~ Ns( age, knots=c(20,40,60,70,80,90) ),
+             family=poisreg, data=subset(Mdm,sex=="M") )
> xf <- glm( cbind(lex.Xst=="Dead",lex.dur)
+               ~ Ns( age, knots=c(20,40,60,70,80,90) ),
+             family=poisreg, data=subset(Mdm,sex=="F") )
> nd <- data.frame( age=seq(10,99,0.5) )
> xpm <- ci.pred( xm, nd )
> xpf <- ci.pred( xf, nd )
> matshade( nd$age, cbind( pm, pf, xpm, xpf )*1000, plot=TRUE,
+            col=c("blue","red"), lwd=2, lty=c(1,1,2,2),
+            log="y", ylim=c(0.5,400), las=1,
+            xlab="Age", ylab="DM mortality per 1000 PY" )
> matpoints( 0:99+0.5,
+             cbind( pmax(astab["M",,"D"]/astab["M",,"Y"],0.00042),
+                    pmax(astab["F",,"D"]/astab["F",,"Y"],0.00045) )*1000,
+             pch=16, col=c("blue","red"), cex=0.4 )
```

CODE EXPLAINED: The outcome is now two columns: the indicator of whether `lex.Xst` is equal to 'Dead' (internally converted from (FALSE/TRUE) to (0/1)), and the risk time in each interval, `lex.dur`. In the dataset `Mdm` the age variable is called `age`, so this must be used in the model as well as in the prediction data frame, here xd. The `matshade` now plots four sets of curves with confidence intervals as semi-transparent shades, with those representing prediction from the disaggregated data as broken lines (`lty=2`). Note that the colours are recycled as blue, red, blue, red for the four different curves. The last `matpoints` function plots the empirical rates in each age class as points, and the rates that are 0 (because of 0 deaths) as 0.42, resp. 0.45, for men and women.

Formally, the two models for DM mortality are slightly different, but conceptually they both represent a set of age-specific rates that varies continuously (smoothly) with age, and which could have generated the observed data. In this sense they both represent a set of *theoretical* rates, as opposed to the *empirical* rates shown as points in Figure 5.2.

5.5.2 Including sex in the model

Instead of modelling rates for men and women separately, we can get the same result by using an interaction model:

```
> mi <- glm( cbind(lex.Xst=="Dead",lex.dur)
+               ~ Ns( age, knots=c(20,40,60,70,80,90) ) * sex,
+             family = poisreg, data = Mdm )
```

This model will give the same fitted values as the separate models for men and women, but it is a bit easier to show the M/W rate ratio from the interaction model:

```
> ndm <- data.frame( age=seq(10,99,0.5), sex="M" )
> ndw <- data.frame( age=seq(10,99,0.5), sex="F" )
> RR <- ci.exp( mi, list( ndm, ndw ) )
```

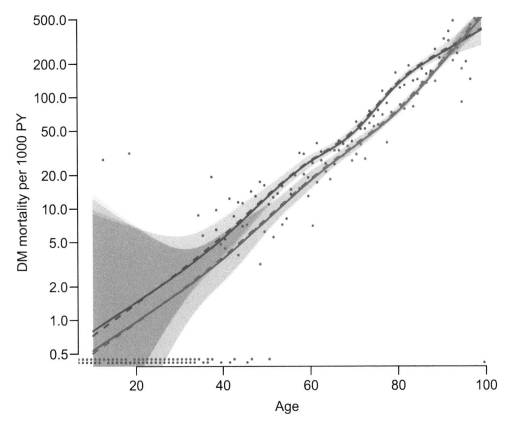

Figure 5.2 Fitted mortality rates for Danish diabetes patients. Full lines are based on 1-year age class tabulated data, broken lines on individually split records. The dots are empirical rates in 1-year classes—rates equal to 0 are indicated just below 0.5 on the y-axis.

```
> matshade( ndm$age, RR, plot=TRUE, lwd=3,
+            ylim=c(0.5,2), log="y",
+            xlab="Age (years)", ylab="M / W rate ratio" )
> abline( h=1 )
```

CODE EXPLAINED: The data frames `ndm` and `ndw` are for predicting mortality rates for men and women, respectively. Entering them in a list as the second argument to `ci.exp` (`list(ndm,ndw)`) will produce the ratio of the two predictions, so the M/W rate ratio as a function of age, which we then can plot with a confidence interval.

The advantage of this is that it is possible to formally test whether there actually is an interaction or if a simple proportional hazards model with a constant M/W rate ratio is adequate:

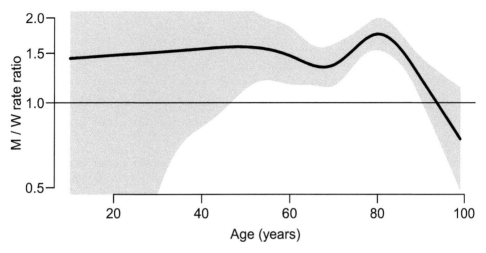

Figure 5.3 Estimated M/W mortality rate ratio by age for Danish diabetes patients. The shaded area represents the 95% confidence interval.

```
> ma <- update( mi, . ~ Ns( age, knots=c(20,40,60,70,80,90) ) + sex )
> anova( ma, mi, test="Chisq" )
Analysis of Deviance Table

Model 1: cbind(lex.Xst == "Dead", lex.dur) ~ Ns(age, knots = c(20, 40,
    60, 70, 80, 90)) + sex
Model 2: cbind(lex.Xst == "Dead", lex.dur) ~ Ns(age, knots = c(20, 40,
    60, 70, 80, 90)) * sex
  Resid. Df Resid. Dev Df Deviance Pr(>Chi)
1     64108      18898
2     64103      18885  5   12.518  0.02834
```

> CODE EXPLAINED: The update function fits a model just as the mi, except for the parts specified. The '. ~' means that the outcome is the same as in mi; only the regression model is different. The model has the same age-effect for men and women, so it assumes a constant M/W rate ratio a cross the age span: a proportional hazards model.

The test (from anova) shows that there is a significant interaction, but the important point is to show how this looks. Figure 5.3 basically shows that the M/W rate ratio is pretty constant till age 80 (at about 1.5) and then declines sharply, so that there is little mortality difference between men and women with diabetes over age 90. Thus there *is* a relevant interaction between sex and age, but it is confined to ages over 80.

5.6 SMR

We may want to compare the mortality rates among diabetes patients to that of the Danish population—a population where we have reliable mortality rates. The mortality rates for the Danish population are available in M.dk:

```
> data( M.dk )
> head( M.dk )
  A sex    P   D        Y      rate
1 0   1 1974 459 35963.33 12.762999
2 0   2 1974 303 34382.83  8.812537
3 0   1 1975 435 36099.00 12.050195
4 0   2 1975 311 34652.17  8.974908
5 0   1 1976 405 34965.00 11.583012
6 0   2 1976 258 33278.33  7.752792
```

We can make a comparison by computing the *expected* number of deaths in the diabetes population under the assumption that the mortality rates were as in the Danish population. If we want to compute the expected number of deaths among the diabetes patients we must take each piece of follow-up among the diabetes patients and multiply its length with the corresponding population mortality rate. This requires that each interval can be matched to the relevant population mortality rate.

If the follow-up interval is small, the expected number is just the probability of death during the interval under the assumption of the population rate being the true mortality. It can be shown that the total (observed) number of deaths divided by the total number of expected deaths is an estimate of the diabetes / population mortality rate ratio, assuming that this is constant. Also it can be shown that the mortality rate ratio can be modelled exactly as the rates by using the expected numbers instead of the person-years in the population.

The population mortality rates in M.dk are classified by sex, age (A), and calendar time (P), so we need the diabetes follow-up classified the same way. In Mdm it is only classified by age, so we must subdivide follow-up by calendar time too:

```
> Mdm <- splitMulti( Mdm, per=1990:2010 )
```

The next step is to match up the population rates from M.dk to the records in Mdm, and compute the expected numbers; to this end we need variables of the same name and type in the two datasets. The intervals of follow-up represented by each record in Mdm do not all start at an integer age or integer year, so we define two variables A and P in Mdm to match the (integer) age and periodclasses in M.dk:

```
> Mdm <- transform( Mdm, A = floor(age), P = floor(per) )
```

> CODE EXPLAINED: transform is used to add new variables to the data frame Mdm, and the function floor rounds to the nearest smaller integer. Thus A and P are integers.

Because Mdm is split by age and per at integer values, no interval extends across either integer age or period, so the classification of follow-up intervals is entirely inside the age-by-period intervals that the population rate M.dk refers to.

We also need the sex variable to match on; this is a factor in Mdm but a numeric variable in M.dk, so we convert the latter to a factor with the same levels as sex in Mdm:

```
> M.dk$sex <- factor( M.dk$sex, labels = c("M","F") )
```

With this in place we can merge the population rates to the diabetes data:

```
> Mxdm <- merge( Mdm, M.dk[,c("sex","A","P","rate")], all.x=TRUE )
> dim(M.dk) ; dim(Mdm) ; dim( Mxdm)
[1] 7800    6
```

```
[1] 114501     15
[1] 114501     16
> Mxdm <- transform( Mxdm, E = lex.dur * rate/1000 )
```

> CODE EXPLAINED: merge joins the two datasets Mdm and M.dk on the common variables, in this case sex, A and P; all.x=TRUE means that all records from Mdm are retained, and that records in M.dk not finding a match are discarded, so effectively we are adding the variable rate from the data frame M.dk. Any record from Mdm that finds no match in M.dk will get a NA for the variable rate.
>
> Finally, we compute the expected number of deaths; the risk time lex.dur is in years, but the rate is in units of 1000 years^{-1}, so we must divide by 1000.

Finally, we can replicate the table of rates from p. 94:

```
> stat.table( index = sex,
+            contents = list( D = sum( lex.Xst=="Dead" ),
+                             Exp = sum( E ),
+                             SMR = ratio( lex.Xst=="Dead", E, 100 ) ),
+            margin = TRUE,
+            data = Mxdm )
 ------------------------------
 sex           D       Exp      SMR
 ------------------------------
 M       1342.00   796.09   168.57
 F       1153.00   747.58   154.23

 Total   2495.00  1543.67   161.63
 ------------------------------
```

> CODE EXPLAINED: The index argument defines the cells of the table, in this case three, one for each sex, plus 1 because we asked for a margin (margin=TRUE). The contents argument defines what goes in each cell of the table, in this case three numbers labelled D, Exp, and SMR. The dataset Mxdm is a Lexis object so deaths are defined by lex.Xst. The expression lex.Xst=="Dead" is a logical indicator of whether a death occurred; E is simply the expected number of deaths in each interval. The ratio of the two is then multiplied by 100 to give the SMR in % as is customary.

From the table we see that men have a slightly higher SMR than women, but primarily we see a general pattern of some 60% higher mortality among diabetes patients relative to the general population.

5.6.1 Modelling the SMR

The table actually shows estimates from two models: one with an overall constant SMR between diabetes patients and population, and one with separate SMRs for men and women. Just as we did for the rates, we can reproduce these by Poisson models:

```
> smr1 <- glm( cbind(lex.Xst=="Dead",E) ~ 1, family=poisreg, data = Mxdm )
> smrx <- update( smr1, . ~ sex - 1 )
> round( rbind( ci.exp( smrx ),
+               ci.exp( smr1 ) ) * 100, 2 )
```

```
            exp(Est.)   2.5%   97.5%
sexM           168.57 159.79 177.84
sexF           154.23 145.58 163.40
(Intercept)    161.63 155.41 168.10
```

> CODE EXPLAINED: The model is precisely as a model for rates, except that the person-years is replaced by the expected numbers, E, as the second column of the response. The first model just estimates an overall SMR, and the second (via update) derives estimates separately for men and women.
>
> The final statement just puts the estimates in the same order as those from stat.table, but here they are with confidence limits.

However, even if the expected numbers are computed from rates matched by age and calendar time, the SMR can depend on age as well.

Thus we can model SMR by age and sex as we did before with the rates:

```
> smra <- glm( cbind(lex.Xst=="Dead", E)
+                  ~ Ns( age, knots=c(20,40,60,70,80,90) ) * sex,
+                  family = poisreg, data = Mxdm )
```

We can use the prediction data frames to produce estimates of SMR by age:

```
>  ndm <- data.frame( age=seq(10,99,0.5), sex="M" )
>  ndw <- data.frame( age=seq(10,99,0.5), sex="F" )
> smrM <- ci.pred( smra, ndm )
> smrW <- ci.pred( smra, ndw )
> matshade( ndm$age, cbind( smrM, smrW), plot=TRUE,
+           col = c("blue","red"), lwd = 3,
+           ylim = c(0.5,10), log = "y",
+           xlab = "Age (years)", ylab = "SMR: DM vs population" )
> abline( h=1 )
```

> CODE EXPLAINED: The data frames ndm and ndw are for predicting the SMR for men and women, respectively. ci.pred produces predicted values from the model, one per record in the data frames ndm and ndw. The resulting SMRs as functions of age are then plotted together with shaded confidence intervals using matshade.

We see from the Figure 5.4 that the SMR decreases by age for both men and women, from about 4–5 at young ages to some 1.5 at age 80, and with no apparent difference between men and women.

Analysis of the SMR (rate ratio relative to the general population) is completely parallel to the analysis of rates; we just replace the person-years with the expected number of deaths. The technical challenge is to get the population rates attached to the follow-up dataset.

Note that there is no formal requirement that the follow-up data be subdivided precisely as the population rate data; the only requirement is that each piece of follow-up can be matched to a population mortality rate.

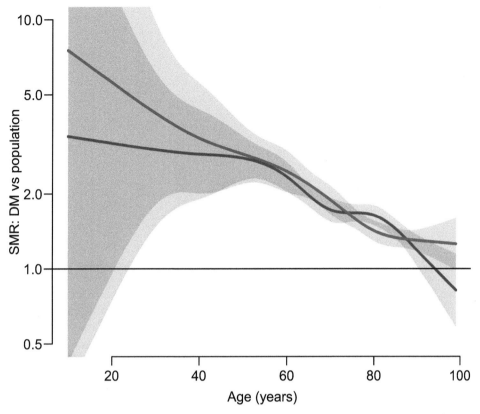

Figure 5.4 Relative mortality (SMR) between DM and the general population (SMR) for men and women. Red curves are women, blue are men, and shaded areas are 95% confidence intervals.

5.7 Time-dependent variables

This is an advanced section that can be skipped at first reading; further details can be found in [4].

5.7.1 *Cutting time at a specific date*

If we have a recording of the date of a specific event as for example recovery or relapse, or as in the diabetes data, the date of the start of insulin therapy, doins, we may classify follow-up time as being before or after this intermediate event.

In data terms this is achieved with the function cutLexis, which has 5 mandatory arguments: the Lexis object, the time of the intermediate event, the time-scale it refers to, the name of the (new) state following the intermediate event, and finally the precursor states (explained below):

```
> Cdm <- cutLexis( data = Ldm,
+                   cut = Ldm$doins,
+             timescale = "per",
+             new.state = "Ins",
+       precursor.states = "Alive" )
> whp <- c(5:6,15,91)
> subset( Cdm, lex.id %in% whp )[,c(1:6,12)]
          age      per  lex.dur lex.Cst lex.Xst lex.id     doins
5     75.77550 2008.653 1.344285   Alive   Alive      5        NA
6     80.01643 2007.886 2.036961   Alive    Dead      6        NA
15    58.13005 2002.550 2.803559   Alive     Ins     15  2005.354
10011 60.93361 2005.354 4.643395     Ins     Ins     15  2005.354
91    69.55784 1998.898 3.162218   Alive     Ins     91  2002.060
10087 72.72005 2002.060 3.304586     Ins    Dead     91  2002.060
```

CODE EXPLAINED: The cutLexis function cuts the follow-up of each person at the dates in the cut argument whose values refer to the time-scale given in the timescale argument. So the variable doins refers to the time-scale per, which is just calendar time coded as years. The new.state gives the name of the state to which persons move at the cut date. The precursor.states argument is explained in detail below.

whp is just a vector of 4 select ids that provide illustrative persons, and so subset restricts to these using the %in% operator (in mathematics known as '∈').

We see that person 15 starts insulin and exits the study on insulin, whereas person 91 also starts insulin, but exits dead some time in 2005 (the value of per (start of last interval) plus lex.dur (length of last interval)).

The same can be done using the split dataset Mdm instead of Ldm:

```
> CMdm <- cutLexis( data = Mdm,
+                   cut = Mdm$doins,
+             timescale = "per",
+             new.state = "Ins",
+       precursor.states = "Alive" )
> subset( CMdm, lex.id %in% whp )[,c(1:6,12)]
     lex.id      age      per   lex.dur lex.Cst lex.Xst     doins
1:        5 75.77550 2008.653 0.22450376   Alive   Alive        NA
2:        5 76.00000 2008.877 0.12251882   Alive   Alive        NA
3:        5 76.12252 2009.000 0.87748118   Alive   Alive        NA
4:        5 77.00000 2009.877 0.11978097   Alive   Alive        NA
5:        6 80.01643 2007.886 0.11362081   Alive   Alive        NA
6:        6 80.13005 2008.000 0.86995209   Alive   Alive        NA
7:        6 81.00000 2008.870 0.13004791   Alive   Alive        NA
8:        6 81.13005 2009.000 0.86995209   Alive   Alive        NA
9:        6 82.00000 2009.870 0.05338809   Alive    Dead        NA
10:      15 58.13005 2002.550 0.44969199   Alive   Alive  2005.354
11:      15 58.57974 2003.000 0.42026010   Alive   Alive  2005.354
12:      15 59.00000 2003.420 0.57973990   Alive   Alive  2005.354
13:      15 59.57974 2004.000 0.42026010   Alive   Alive  2005.354
14:      15 60.00000 2004.420 0.57973990   Alive   Alive  2005.354
15:      15 60.57974 2005.000 0.35386721   Alive     Ins  2005.354
16:      15 60.93361 2005.354 0.06639288     Ins     Ins  2005.354
17:      15 61.00000 2005.420 0.57973990     Ins     Ins  2005.354
```

```
18:     15 61.57974 2006.000 0.42026010    Ins    Ins 2005.354
19:     15 62.00000 2006.420 0.57973990    Ins    Ins 2005.354
20:     15 62.57974 2007.000 0.42026010    Ins    Ins 2005.354
21:     15 63.00000 2007.420 0.57973990    Ins    Ins 2005.354
22:     15 63.57974 2008.000 0.42026010    Ins    Ins 2005.354
23:     15 64.00000 2008.420 0.57973990    Ins    Ins 2005.354
24:     15 64.57974 2009.000 0.42026010    Ins    Ins 2005.354
25:     15 65.00000 2009.420 0.57700205    Ins    Ins 2005.354
26:     91 69.55784 1998.898 0.10198494  Alive  Alive 2002.060
27:     91 69.65982 1999.000 0.34017796  Alive  Alive 2002.060
28:     91 70.00000 1999.340 0.65982204  Alive  Alive 2002.060
29:     91 70.65982 2000.000 0.34017796  Alive  Alive 2002.060
30:     91 71.00000 2000.340 0.65982204  Alive  Alive 2002.060
31:     91 71.65982 2001.000 0.34017796  Alive  Alive 2002.060
32:     91 72.00000 2001.340 0.65982204  Alive  Alive 2002.060
33:     91 72.65982 2002.000 0.06023272  Alive    Ins 2002.060
34:     91 72.72005 2002.060 0.27994524    Ins    Ins 2002.060
35:     91 73.00000 2002.340 0.65982204    Ins    Ins 2002.060
36:     91 73.65982 2003.000 0.34017796    Ins    Ins 2002.060
37:     91 74.00000 2003.340 0.65982204    Ins    Ins 2002.060
38:     91 74.65982 2004.000 0.34017796    Ins    Ins 2002.060
39:     91 75.00000 2004.340 0.65982204    Ins    Ins 2002.060
40:     91 75.65982 2005.000 0.34017796    Ins    Ins 2002.060
41:     91 76.00000 2005.340 0.02464066    Ins   Dead 2002.060
     lex.id      age      per  lex.dur lex.Cst lex.Xst    doins
```

Thus *splitting* follow-up at prespecified points on a time-scale and *cutting* follow-up at the time of an intermediate event are interchangeable; the resulting objects will be identical.

The precursor states

Note that follow-up subsequent to the intermediate event (initiation of insulin, at doins) is classified in lex.Cst as being in state Ins, but that the final transition to Dead' is preserved (person with lex.id 91). This is the point of the precursor.states= argument: it names the states (in this case Alive) that will be over-ridden by new.state (in this case Ins). Clearly, the state Dead should not be updated even if it is after the time where the persons moves to state Ins. In other words, only state Alive is a precursor to state Ins; state Dead is always subsequent to state Ins. This is the reason that the precursor.states= is needed as an argument to cutLexis; the last record of persons 15 and 91 are treated differently: person 15 ends Alive (a precursor state) and so stays as Ins, whereas person 91 ends as Dead and therefore moves from Ins to Dead at the end.

5.7.2 Modelling time-dependent variables

Once the split data have been subdivided by (current) state, recorded in the variable lex.Cst, this can be used as a covariate; the effect of lex.Cst=="Ins" will show the effect of beginning insulin treatment—or more precisely, the effect of being on insulin treatment.

```
> xmv <- glm( cbind(lex.Xst=="Dead", lex.dur)
+            ~ Ns( age, knots=c(20,40,60,70,80,90) ) + lex.Cst,
+            family = poisreg,
```

```
+                   data = subset(CMdm,sex=="M") )
> ci.exp( xmv, subset="Cst" )
             exp(Est.)      2.5%      97.5%
lex.CstIns   2.150278  1.873953  2.467349
```

> CODE EXPLAINED: The only difference to the previous model is that we added `lex.Cst`
> to the predictor; the estimate (extracted by `ci.exp`) is 2.15, meaning that a person on
> insulin (at any age) has a 2.15 times larger mortality than a person of the same age not
> on insulin.

The effect of insulin here cannot be interpreted as the insulin effect; it is *confounded by
indication*: persons are not randomized til insulin. They are put on insulin treatment for a
reason. So the 2.15 is the combined effect of being a person needing insulin therapy and
the effect of insulin. Most likely the first carries a larger relative risk than 2.15, but no data
are available to corroborate this:

```
> ndA <- data.frame( age = seq(10,99,0.5), lex.Cst = "Alive" )
> ndI <- transform( ndA, lex.Cst = ifelse(age>=60, "Ins", NA) )
> pmA <- ci.pred( xmv, ndA )
> pmI <- ci.pred( xmv, ndI )
> matshade( nd$age, cbind( pmA, pmI )*1000, plot=TRUE,
+           col = c("blue","orange"), lwd = 2, lty = 1,
+           log = "y", ylim = c(0.5,400)*2, las = 1,
+           xlab = "Age", ylab = "DM mortality per 1000 PY" )
> abline( v = 60, lty = 3 )
```

> CODE EXPLAINED: We devise two prediction frames, `ndA` for a person not on insulin (in state
> 'Alive'), and one `ndI` for a person on insulin from age 60 with the missing value of the
> variable `lex.Cst` before age 60. We make predictions `pmA` and `pmI` using `ci.pred` and
> plot these. Note that the `ndI` has missing values and so produces a prediction with NAs
> for ages under 60.
>   `matshade` therefore produces lines for the entire agespan corresponding to the
> mortality among men not on insulin (from `pmA`), but only for ages over 60 for persons
> on insulin, illustrating the estimated jump in mortality at the time of insulin start.

From Figure 5.5 we clearly see that the model is a *proportional hazards model*; the mortality
rates in persons on and not on insulin are assumed to have the same shape. Since the
y-axis is logarithmic this shows up as parallel curves.

Survival?

We may want to derive the survival function (the probability of surviving *t*) of a person say
aged 50 from the estimated mortality rates. This would, however, not be possible based on
the model we fitted for a person not on insulin. If we were to use the mortality rate derived
for a person not on insulin, we would be referring to a situation where the occurrence 'start
of insulin' was not possible.

But it *would* be possible to derive a valid survival function for a person on insulin at, say,
age 60. This is because there is only one possible exit from the `Ins` state, namely `Death`.
These issues are further discussed in Chapter 8 on survival.

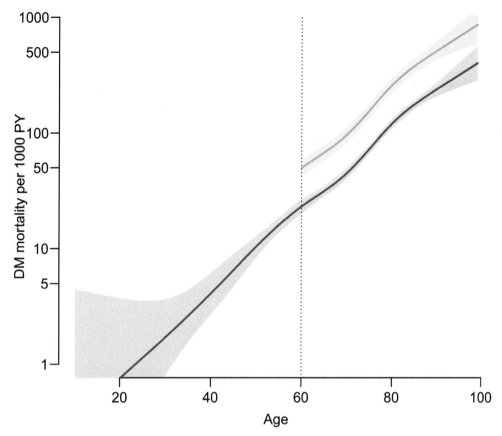

Figure 5.5 Predicted mortality rates for Danish male diabetes patients. The blue line is for men not on insulin; the orange line is for men on insulin.

5.7.3 *Clinical measurements in cohort studies*

Some cohort studies have follow-up visits where clinical measurements (such as blood pressure, weight, or cholesterol levels) are taken. If we want to assess the effect of such clinical variables we must amend the dataset so that each time of follow-up has the value of the most recent clinical measurement.

This means that we must cut the follow-up at the time of clinical visit and assign clinical measurement values to the follow-up after the visit. If more than one visit is made by a person, clinical values are replaced by the most recent ones. The values for the clinical variables will be missing (NA) for any follow-up time prior to the first visit.

Here is a small artificial example that illustrates the machinery that attaches clinical measurements to a Lexis data frame of follow-up:

```
> clin <- data.frame( lex.id = c( 6, 6,15,15,91),
+                         ex = c("one","two")[c(1,2,1,2,2)],
+                        per = c(2008.1,2009.1,2003.8,2007.2,2003.1),
+                        sbp = c(120,134,149,166,120),
+                         wt = c(90,93,107,103,75) )
> clin
```

```
  lex.id   ex    per sbp  wt
1      6  one 2008.1 120  90
2      6  two 2009.1 134  93
3     15  one 2003.8 149 107
4     15  two 2007.2 166 103
5     91  two 2003.1 120  75
> Zdm <- subset( CMdm, lex.id %in% c(6,15,91) )[,1:6]
```

clin is a data frame with one or more clinical measurements at given dates (per) for the persons 6, 15, and 91. Zdm is a subset of the data frame CMdm with only records for persons 6, 15, and 91.

```
> Kdm <- addCov.Lexis( Zdm,          # Lexis data frame to be expanded
+                      clin,          # data frame with id, date and measures
+                timescale = "per",# time scale variable
+                   exnam = "ex", # exam name variable
+                addScales = TRUE )
> od <- options(digits=5)
>       Kdm[,c(timeScales(Kdm),"lex.dur")] <-
+ round( Kdm[,c(timeScales(Kdm),"lex.dur")], 2 )
> Kdm[,c("lex.id",timeScales(Kdm)[-1],
+        "lex.dur","lex.Cst","lex.Xst","ex","sbp","wt")]
```

	lex.id	per	tfone	tftwo	tfc	lex.dur	lex.Cst	lex.Xst	ex	sbp	wt
32	6	2007.9	NA	NA	Inf	0.11	Alive	Alive	<NA>	NA	NA
33	6	2008.0	NA	NA	Inf	0.10	Alive	Alive	<NA>	NA	NA
35	6	2008.1	0.00	NA	0.00	0.77	Alive	Alive	one	120	90
37	6	2008.9	0.77	NA	0.77	0.13	Alive	Alive	one	120	90
38	6	2009.0	0.90	NA	0.90	0.10	Alive	Alive	one	120	90
40	6	2009.1	1.00	0.00	0.00	0.77	Alive	Alive	two	134	93
42	6	2009.9	1.77	0.77	0.77	0.05	Alive	Dead	two	134	93
11	15	2002.5	NA	NA	Inf	0.45	Alive	Alive	<NA>	NA	NA
12	15	2003.0	NA	NA	Inf	0.42	Alive	Alive	<NA>	NA	NA
16	15	2003.4	NA	NA	Inf	0.38	Alive	Alive	<NA>	NA	NA
17	15	2003.8	0.00	NA	0.00	0.20	Alive	Alive	one	149	107
18	15	2004.0	0.20	NA	0.20	0.42	Alive	Alive	one	149	107
21	15	2004.4	0.62	NA	0.62	0.58	Alive	Alive	one	149	107
22	15	2005.0	1.20	NA	1.20	0.35	Alive	Ins	one	149	107
25	15	2005.3	1.55	NA	1.55	0.07	Ins	Ins	one	149	107
26	15	2005.4	1.62	NA	1.62	0.58	Ins	Ins	one	149	107
27	15	2006.0	2.20	NA	2.20	0.42	Ins	Ins	one	149	107
28	15	2006.4	2.62	NA	2.62	0.58	Ins	Ins	one	149	107
29	15	2007.0	3.20	NA	3.20	0.20	Ins	Ins	one	149	107
30	15	2007.2	3.40	0.00	0.00	0.22	Ins	Ins	two	166	103
31	15	2007.4	3.62	0.22	0.22	0.58	Ins	Ins	two	166	103
34	15	2008.0	4.20	0.80	0.80	0.42	Ins	Ins	two	166	103
36	15	2008.4	4.62	1.22	1.22	0.58	Ins	Ins	two	166	103
39	15	2009.0	5.20	1.80	1.80	0.42	Ins	Ins	two	166	103
41	15	2009.4	5.62	2.22	2.22	0.58	Ins	Ins	two	166	103
1	91	1998.9	NA	NA	Inf	0.10	Alive	Alive	<NA>	NA	NA
2	91	1999.0	NA	NA	Inf	0.34	Alive	Alive	<NA>	NA	NA
3	91	1999.3	NA	NA	Inf	0.66	Alive	Alive	<NA>	NA	NA
4	91	2000.0	NA	NA	Inf	0.34	Alive	Alive	<NA>	NA	NA
5	91	2000.3	NA	NA	Inf	0.66	Alive	Alive	<NA>	NA	NA

```
6      91 2001.0    NA    NA   Inf   0.34   Alive   Alive  <NA>   NA   NA
7      91 2001.3    NA    NA   Inf   0.66   Alive   Alive  <NA>   NA   NA
8      91 2002.0    NA    NA   Inf   0.06   Alive     Ins  <NA>   NA   NA
9      91 2002.1    NA    NA   Inf   0.28     Ins     Ins  <NA>   NA   NA
10     91 2002.3    NA    NA   Inf   0.66     Ins     Ins  <NA>   NA   NA
13     91 2003.0    NA    NA   Inf   0.10     Ins     Ins  <NA>   NA   NA
14     91 2003.1    NA  0.00 0.00   0.24     Ins     Ins   two  120   75
15     91 2003.3    NA  0.24 0.24   0.66     Ins     Ins   two  120   75
19     91 2004.0    NA  0.90 0.90   0.34     Ins     Ins   two  120   75
20     91 2004.3    NA  1.24 1.24   0.66     Ins     Ins   two  120   75
23     91 2005.0    NA  1.90 1.90   0.34     Ins     Ins   two  120   75
24     91 2005.3    NA  2.24 2.24   0.02     Ins    Dead   two  120   75
> timeSince( Kdm )
  age    per tfone tftwo    tfc
   ""     ""  "one" "two"     ""
> options( od )
```

CODE EXPLAINED: clin is just a made-up example data frame with measurements of blood pressure (sbp, mmHg) and weight (wt, kg) on three persons, lex.id 6, 15, and 91, at two different rounds (one, two).

We want to add these measurements to the corresponding subset of 3 persons from CMdm—subsetted to (Zdm).

The options is just to set the number of significant digits to print so we get a slightly more compact print. Assignment to an object enables an easy way of resetting to previous values.

For printing, we round the time-scales and the lex.dur variable, and then select the relevant variables from Kdm using '[,]' with the variable names after the comma. We use timeSince to list the variables that have time-scale status, as well as the events that make up the origin of the time-scales.

We see that we have created 3 new time-scales: time since examination rounds one (tfone) and two (tftwo), and time since the latest (tfc). Note that tfc is not a proper time-scale because it jumps back at every new clinical measurement, so it cannot be used to calculate risk time like the other time-scales.

Also note that the behaviour of addCov is to carry the last clinical observation forward, so the resulting Lexis object has both the most recent clinical measurement and the time since it was taken.

Analysis using clinical measurements

When using the most recent clinical measurements in the analysis of rates, the analysis will be using what is normally termed 'updated values' of the clinical measurements. This type of analysis is aimed at quantifying the effects of the clinical measurements on some type of event occurrence. Some datasets, primarily those from population-based studies with widely spaced examinations, will have few measurements per person, whereas others, primarily those based on clinical routine records for patients, will have many measurements per person.

An underlying assumption is almost always that the clinical measurements represent the clinical status of each person at the time of follow-up. This is presumably a reasonable assumption shortly after the time of measurement, but less likely the longer time has passed since the measurement. Another way of putting this is that an 'old' clinical measurement represents a current clinical status with increasing uncertainty as time goes by, so the natural expectation would be that the predictive value of a measurement decrease by time. Model-wise this would would be captured by an interaction between the measurement and the time since measurement. This would allow the effect to decay from the time of measurement.

The models used for assessing the effects of updated clinical measurements will not be suitable for predicting occurrence rates, because the models will be *conditional* on the values of the clinical measurements, and therefore a probability model for time development of all clinical variables will be needed in order to derive predicted rates.

There is a theory and a corresponding modelling machinery that allows simultaneous modelling of both the event outcome and the clinical measurements; it goes by the name of 'joint modelling'. This is another topic which is outside the scope of this book.

CHAPTER 6

Parametrization and prediction of rates

This section gives an overview of parametrizing quantitative covariate effects, that is, describing how variables (covariates) influence the outcome variable, be that disease odds, rates, or some quantitative measurement.

6.1 Predictions and contrasts

When reporting rate ratios between two groups or the odds ratio of a disease associated with a certain difference in exposure we are using *contrasts* of the outcome variable between different values of a covariate to describe the effect. Thus we use ratios or differences, the former dimensionless, the latter with the same dimension as the outcome.

But when reporting the mortality rate in, say, 60-year-old males we are making a *prediction* of the outcome. This requires a set of values for *all* covariates in a model. This is opposed to the *contrasts*, such as the M/W rate ratio, where only covariates involved in a given contrast need to be specified.

In both cases we are reporting functions of the parameters in the model; contrasts typically only involve a subset of the parameters, whereas predictions necessarily use the values for *all* of them.

When describing the effects of covariates by a model we normally use a *linear predictor*, i.e. a linear combination of (functions of) covariate values for individual i in the study:

$$\eta_i = \sum_j \beta_j x_{ij}$$

Here the *x*es are the variables that enter directly in the linear predictor; x_{ij} is the value of the jth variable for the ith person. The *x*es are not necessarily identical to actually measured covariates in a study—often a measured covariate will be represented by several variables, for example factor level indicators for a categorical covariate, or the measured value of a quantitative variable and one or more mathematical functions of it (such as x^2).

Note that there is nothing that formally bars us from specifying non-linear functions of variables and parameters in a model. But the linear formulation above is very flexible and easy to work with, so really mostly used out of computational convenience.

6.2 Prediction of a single rate

Here we use the `diet` data, and use simple estimation of rates, as first described in section 2.2 on p. 42.

Epidemiology with R. Bendix Carstensen, Oxford University Press (2021). © Bendix Carstensen.
DOI: 10.1093/oso/9780198841326.003.0007

If we use the diet data and estimate the overall rate of CHD, we are essentially assuming a model with constant mortality rate. The maximum likelihood estimator of the rate is D/Y, the number of events divided by the total risk time (person-years), and the standard error of the log rate is $1/\sqrt{D}$, so we can construct the estimate and the confidence interval:

```
> data( diet )
> attach( diet )
> y <- cal.yr(dox) - cal.yr(doe)   # Follow-up time in years for each
                                     person
> Y <- sum( y )                    # Total no. person-years
> D <- sum( chd )                  # Total no. of CHD events
> rate <- D / Y
> erf <- exp( 1.96 / sqrt( D ) )   # Error-factor
> c( rate, rate / erf, rate * erf )
[1] 0.009992031 0.007484256 0.013340094
```

> CODE EXPLAINED: data gets the data frame diet from the Epi package, whereas attach places it in the search-path so we directly can access the variables in the data frame.
>
> The variable dox and doe are date variables (try str(diet)), so stored in units of days. cal.yr transforms a date variable to units of years so we can compute the follow-up time in years, by transforming to years before subtracting entry date from exit date.
>
> Here we have used the formula for computation of the confidence interval based on the normal approximation to the log rate.

The likelihood for a constant rate based on D events and Y risk time is proportional to a Poisson likelihood for the observation D with mean λY, where λ is the rate. Hence we can estimate the rate using a Poisson model. In the model we need the log of the follow-up time for each person as the offset variable:

```
> m1 <- glm( chd ~ 1, offset = log(y), family = poisson )
> round( ci.lin(m1, Exp = TRUE), 3 )
           Estimate StdErr     z P exp(Est.)  2.5% 97.5%
(Intercept)  -4.606  0.147 -31.24 0      0.01 0.007 0.013
> ci.exp(m1)
              exp(Est.)        2.5%       97.5%
(Intercept) 0.009992031 0.007484355 0.01333992
```

> CODE EXPLAINED: glm with family=poisson fits a Poisson model, here with one parameter, the intercept (called '1'), while including the log-person-time as a covariate with a fixed coefficient of 1; this is what is called an offset.
>
> The function ci.lin from the Epi package takes the parameter(s) from a model and displays them with confidence limits, and the Exp=TRUE option requests that the exponential of the estimates and corresponding confidence intervals be computed, which gives exactly the confidence intervals we obtained 'by hand' before. A convenient wrapper is ci.exp that only gives the exponentiated parameter with confidence interval (which is what you normally want when modelling rates).

Normally we would want the rates in units per 1000 person-years or something similar, which is most conveniently done by scaling the ys when fitting the model:

```
> m1 <- glm(chd ~ 1, offset = log(y/1000), family = poisson)
> round( ci.exp(m1), 2 )
            exp(Est.) 2.5% 97.5%
(Intercept)      9.99 7.48 13.34
```

The offset machinery is a bit awkward; it comes from the identity of the rate likelihood and the Poisson likelihood. It is more intuitive to use the `poisreg` family where the response variable is a two-column vector of events and person-time—the two components of the response for a rate outcome:

```
> m2 <- glm( cbind(chd, y/1000) ~ 1, family = poisreg )
> round( ci.exp( m2 ), 2 )
            exp(Est.) 2.5% 97.5%
(Intercept)      9.99 7.48 13.34
```

> CODE EXPLAINED: When using the `poisreg` family, the response (l.h.s. of the '~') must be a two-column matrix with the first column holding the event indicator (a count) and the second the person-time. Here this is done by using `cbind` to bind the vector of events (chd) and the vector of person-time in 1000s (y/1000) together to a two-column matrix. The r.h.s. of the model formula is just 1, so an overall rate is estimated.

A side effect of using `poisreg` is that the fitting of the models is slightly faster, but this is only tangible for very large datasets.

6.3 Categorical variables

6.3.1 *Groups and rate ratios*

If we want to estimate the rates separately in different groups of persons (occupational groups, for example) we can compute the rates in the groups separately—note that the code is much the same as before, except we are now referring to vectors instead of scalars:

```
> st <- stat.table( index = job,
+             contents = list(D=sum(chd),
+                             Y=sum(y),
+                          rate=ratio(chd,y,1000)),
+             margins = TRUE,
+                 data = diet )
> print( st, digits = c(sum=0, ratio=2) )
-----------------------------------
job              D     Y    rate
-----------------------------------
Driver          12  1227    9.78
Conductor       14  1043   13.42
Bank worker     20  2333    8.57

Total           46  4604    9.99
-----------------------------------
```

```
> D <- st[1,]
> Y <- st[2,]
> rate <- D/Y * 1000
> erf <- exp( 1.96 / sqrt( D ) ) # Error-factor
> round( cbind( D, Y, rate, rate/erf, rate * erf ), 2 )
               D      Y  rate
Driver        12 1227.10  9.78  5.55 17.22
Conductor     14 1043.45 13.42  7.95 22.65
Bank worker   20 2333.12  8.57  5.53 13.29
Total         46 4603.67  9.99  7.48 13.34
```

indexing

> CODE EXPLAINED: `stat.table` produces a table classified by the variables in the `index` argument. Each cell in the table (in this case one for each level of `job`) can have several entries, in this case the sum of the CHD events, the sum of the person-years, and the ratio of these scaled by 1000. There is a `print` method for `stat.table` that allows control over the number of digits printed.
>
> The result is an array, a multidimensional structure classified by the `contents` plus the elements in `index`. In this case a 2-dimensional structure, so the first two elements of the first dimension will be events and person-years, classified by `job`—including the total (requested by `margins=TRUE`). So D is the number of CVD events, Y the person-years, both vectors of length 4; 3 categories of `job` plus the total. The empirical rates and corresponding confidence intervals are computed according to the formulae based on the normal approximation to the distribution of the log rate, formula (5.2), p. 97.

The rate ratio between two of the occupational groups, e.g. conductors and bank workers, and the corresponding confidence interval can also be computed 'by hand':

```
> RR <- rate[2] / rate[3]
> erf.RR <- exp( 1.96 * sqrt( sum(1/D[2:3]) ) ) # Error-factor
> round( setNames( c( RR, RR/erf.RR, RR*erf.RR),
+                  c("RR",     "lo",      "hi") ), 2 )
  RR   lo   hi
1.57 0.79 3.10
```

> CODE EXPLAINED: The vector `rate` holds the rates for the three job categories, so here we take the ratio of the 2th to the 3rd.
>
> The rest is just using the standard formulae (Eq. (5.3), p. 97) for the confidence interval of a rate ratio; note that `1/D[2:3]` is a vector of length 2, with elements equal to the inverse of the 2nd and the 3rd elements of D. The `setNames` function puts names on the entries of a vector, so the printed results becomes human readable.

The rate ratio is 1.57, but the confidence interval is (0.79–3.10), so we have very little information about the rate ratio, and only weak evidence that the rate among condutors is higher than among bank workers. On the other hand, the data are also compatible with a 3 times higher mortality among conductors relative to bank workers.

As before, the underlying model is one with constant rates, now separately in three groups, and the rates can therefore be computed using a Poisson model. Here we rescale the person-years, y, by 1000 so that we get rates in units of events per 1000:

```
> m2a <- glm( cbind(chd,y/1000) ~ job     , family=poisreg, data=diet )
> round( ci.exp( m2a ), 2 )
                  exp(Est.) 2.5% 97.5%
(Intercept)            9.78 5.55 17.22
jobConductor           1.37 0.63  2.97
jobBank worker         0.88 0.43  1.79
> m2b <- glm( cbind(chd,y/1000) ~ job - 1, family=poisreg, data=diet )
> round( ci.exp( m2b ), 2 )
                  exp(Est.) 2.5% 97.5%
jobDriver              9.78 5.55 17.22
jobConductor          13.42 7.95 22.65
jobBank worker         8.57 5.53 13.29
```

CODE EXPLAINED: The two models fitted are identical, and only the *parametrization* is different; the first, m2a, is parametrized by the rate in group 1 and the rate ratios of the two other groups relative to the first, whereas the second model, m2b, is parametrized by the three rates—the '-1' removes the intercept from the model, and therefore uses indicators of all three groups as covariates.

Comparing all groups

ci.exp (and ci.lin) has a built-in facility that returns all contrasts between factor levels—it requires the subset argument to return sane results:

```
> round( ci.exp( m2b, subset='job', diff=TRUE ), 2 )
                           exp(Est.) 2.5% 97.5%
Driver vs. Conductor            0.73 0.34  1.58
Driver vs. Bank worker          1.14 0.56  2.33
Conductor vs. Bank worker       1.57 0.79  3.10
```

Subsetting with a name of a factor (here job) will give the same result used on the two models m2a and m2b; this is not the case if subsetting is by a numerical vector.

In fact all pairwise differences between pairs of any set of parameters in a model can be computed, and ordering matters:

```
> round( ci.exp( m2b, subset=1:3, diff=TRUE ), 2 )
                           exp(Est.) 2.5% 97.5%
Driver vs. Conductor            0.73 0.34  1.58
Driver vs. Bank worker          1.14 0.56  2.33
Conductor vs. Bank worker       1.57 0.79  3.10
> round( ci.exp( m2b, subset=3:1, diff=TRUE ), 2 )
                           exp(Est.) 2.5% 97.5%
Bank worker vs. Conductor       0.64 0.32  1.26
Bank worker vs. Driver          0.88 0.43  1.79
Conductor vs. Driver            1.37 0.63  2.97
```

From these calculations we see that there is no evidence of rates being different between the three occupational groups, which can also be seen using the anova function:

```
> anova( m2a, test="Chisq" )
Analysis of Deviance Table
Model: poisson, link: log
Response: cbind(chd, y/1000)
Terms added sequentially (first to last)


      Df Deviance Resid. Df Resid. Dev Pr(>Chi)
NULL                    336     262.82
job    2   1.6053       334     261.22   0.4481
> anova( m2b, test="Chisq" )
Analysis of Deviance Table
Model: poisson, link: log
Response: cbind(chd, y/1000)
Terms added sequentially (first to last)


      Df Deviance Resid. Df Resid. Dev  Pr(>Chi)
NULL                    337     391.79
job    3  130.58        334     261.22 < 2.2e-16
```

CODE EXPLAINED: The results from the anova depends on the parametrization of the model; using model m2a gives the test of equality of the three rates, i.e. whether the two contrasts are 0; using model m2b gives the test of whether the log of the three rates are all 0, that is, whether the rates all are 1/1000 PY. The latter test is nonsense; the hypothesis depends on the scale chosen for the rates.

Try to re-fit model m2b using rates per 100 instead of per 1000 PY and see what happens when using anova.

The model m2a used for describing rates by a reference rate and a rate ratio is an example of the default *treatment contrasts* that R uses for parametrizing factor effects: a reference level is chosen (defaults to the first level of the factor, in this case Driver), and the response at this level is estimated along with the contrasts between the other factor levels and the reference level.

6.4 Modelling the effect of quantitative variables

If we want to assess the effect of a quantitative variable on an epidemiological response, a natural assumption supporting a causality interpretation would be to assume what Austin Bradford Hill termed a biological gradient [6]:

(5) *Biological gradient:* Fifthly, if the association is one which can reveal a biological gradient, or dose-response curve, then we should look most carefully for such evidence. For instance, the fact that the death rate from cancer of the lung rises linearly with the number of cigarettes smoked daily, adds a very great deal to the simpler evidence that cigarette smokers have a higher death rate than non-smokers.

The mathematical translation of this is that any (small) increase in exposure (the quantitative variable, smoking exposure) entails a (small) increase in the response (lung cancer mortality). Another way of formulating this is to say that we use the information that age, energy intake, or amount of tobacco smoked is a *quantitative* variable and therefore we should expect the effect of it to be a smooth continuous function of it. A linear relationship is just the smoothest possible quantitative relationship.

6.4.1 *Categorizing quantitative variables: don't*

One possibility often used is to group a quantitative variable in intervals and model the effect of it as a factor. This is not advisable because we will (among other things):

- Abandon the ordering of the categories and thus not use the quantitative nature of the variable; and
- Make unrealistic claims that effects are constant in intervals and have abrupt jumps (either way) at cut-points.

Alone on these two grounds, categorizing variables for anything but exploratory purposes should be avoided.

Vanderbilt University's Department of Biostatistics (Nashville, TN, USA) has compiled a comprehensive list of reasons and more details on why not to categorize quantitative variables which is included as Chapter 9.

6.4.2 *Linear effect*

We shall illustrate the point made by Bradford Hill by looking at modelling incidence rates of testis cancer in Denmark in the age span 15–65, available in the data frame `testisDK` in the `Epi` package.

In this dataset the age variable A refers to 1-year ageclasses and the calendar time variable P to calendar years (period). We regard A and P as quantitative variables; the persons in age class a, say, are on average $a + \frac{1}{2}$ years old and the follow-up in calendar year p is on average at date $p + \frac{1}{2}$ (using the convention that $p = 2003.0$ refers to 1 January 2003):

```
> library( Epi )
> data( testisDK )
> tdk <- subset( testisDK, A>14 & A<65 )
> tdk <- transform( tdk, A = A+1/2, P=P+1/2 )
> head( tdk, 4 )
       A      P D        Y
16  15.5 1943.5 0 31188.00
17  16.5 1943.5 0 31654.33
18  17.5 1943.5 0 32084.33
19  18.5 1943.5 0 32681.67
```

CODE EXPLAINED: The `subset` function restricts the data frame to those in ages 15 through 64; `transform` allows redefinition of variables (and construction of new); `head` just lists the first few lines of the data frame `tdk`.

```
> m1 <- glm( cbind(D, Y/10^5) ~ A, family=poisreg, data=tdk )
> round( ci.exp( m1, pval=TRUE ), 3 )
            exp(Est.)   2.5%  97.5% P
(Intercept)    14.605 13.754 15.508 0
A               0.989  0.988  0.991 0
```

> CODE EXPLAINED: The glm with the poisreg family models the rates as derived from D (number of incident cases) and Y (amount of risk time or person-years). Note that we enter the risk time in units of 100,000 years, because we want to model the rates *per* 100,000 PY.
>   ci.exp extracts the estimates and exponentiates them to show rates on this scale as well as the rate ratio associated with age.

The interpretation of the age-effect in this simple model is that the incidence rate of testis cancer changes by a factor 0.989 for each year of age, i.e. a decrease of 1.1% per year of age.

The model is a *linear* model for the log incidence rates; the assumption of linearity implies that regardless of whether we consider the age difference between 26 and 25 or between 58 and 57 of age, the rate ratio is 0.989. Incidentally, the fit of the model is appallingly bad as we shall see.

Note that the *scale* of the (exponentiated) intercept is now an incidence rate, but referring to the incidence rate of testis cancer at age 0—quite an irrelevant quantity. We can re-fit the model by *centring* the age around some sensible age, 30 years, say:

```
> m1c <- glm( cbind(D,Y/10^5) ~ I(A-30), family=poisreg, data=tdk )
> round( ci.exp( m1c ), 3 )
            exp(Est.)   2.5%  97.5%
(Intercept)    10.578 10.334 10.828
I(A - 30)       0.989  0.988  0.991
```

> CODE EXPLAINED: In the specification we used the function I, which prevents the interpretation of its argument as part of the model formula, so that the variable A-30 is used. Had we entered A-30 directly, R would interpret -30 as an attempt to remove the variable 30 from the model. Since '30' is not a valid variable name we would get an error. The I function should be used whenever we want to include arithmetic expressions of variables in a model.

We see that the slope estimate is still the same, but the intercept estimate is now an incidence rate of 10.6 cases per 100,000 PY, referring to the predicted incidence rates at age 30.

Note that we centred the age (A) variable at a nice round number (30 years), which has the effect of rendering the intercept a quantity that can be reasonably communicated. Using the arithmetic mean of age or the median age would make the intercept difficult to communicate. The recommendation is to centre a variable at a nice round and, if possible, subject-matter sensible value of the variable. Note that centring a variable does not change the effect estimate for the variable; it changes the value and interpretation of the *intercept* in the model. The model fit remains the same.

Predicting the rates

We have fitted a model that predicts the incidence rates of testis cancer in Denmark as a function of age. The model is one that describes the log (the link function) of the incidence rate as a linear function of age. We can compute the predicted rate for a select set of values of the explanatory variable A by setting up a *prediction data frame* with a column for each explanatory variable (in this case only one, A), and a row for each point where we want a prediction. Using this as the `newdata` argument to the function `ci.pred` will compute the predicted rates with confidence intervals:

```
> nd <- data.frame( A=seq(15,65,0.5) )
> pr <- ci.pred( m1c, newdata=nd )
> with( tdk, plot( A, D/Y*10^5, pch=16, cex=0.4, col="gray", log="y" ) )
> matshade( nd$A, pr, plot=FALSE, lwd=2 )
```

> CODE EXPLAINED: `nd` is a data frame with one column for each explanatory variable in the model (in this case only one). This is what is required as the `newdata` argument to `ci.pred`, which computes the predicted values on the outcome scale (in this case incidence rates per 100,000 person-years because the second column of the response in the `glm` was in units of 100,000 person-years). `ci.pred` returns a 3-column matrix, with the same number of rows as `nd`, and columns representing estimates and lower and upper (95%) confidence limits.
>
> We then plot the empirical incidence rates using variables from the data frame `tdk` (using the `with` function), with filled points (`pch=16`), of size 0.4 (`cex=0.4`) in grey colour. The *y*-axis is set up as a logarithmic axis using `log="y"`.
>
> The function `matshade` takes an *x*-vector as first argument and a matrix of 3 (or a multiple of 3) columns as argument (containing estimate, lower and upper confidence limits), and produces a plot with a shaded area for the confidence interval, and since `plot=FALSE` the graph is added to the existing plot. `lwd=2` makes the line 2 pixels wide.

Of course, the assumption of a simple linear relationship between age and log-incidence rates is grossly inadequate as a description of the age-effect on testis cancer incidence rates in Denmark (Figure 6.1).

6.4.3 *Polynomial effects*

The linearity assumption implies that the effect of age is the same across the age range. We can make a simple extension of the model that relaxes this assumption by including an effect of the square of age. The model will still be a linear model in the sense that we still have a linear predictor. The non-linear effect of age comes about because both A and A^2 are included as covariates:

```
> m2 <- glm( cbind(D,Y/10^5) ~ A + I(A^2), family=poisreg, data=tdk )
> round( ci.lin( m2 ), 4 )
            Estimate StdErr        z P    2.5%    97.5%
(Intercept)  -1.3622 0.1114 -12.2308 0 -1.5805  -1.1439
A             0.2301 0.0062  36.9017 0  0.2179   0.2423
I(A^2)       -0.0032 0.0001 -38.5854 0 -0.0034  -0.0030
```

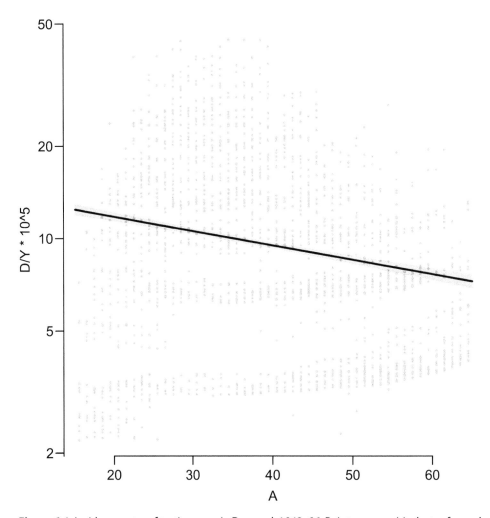

Figure 6.1 Incidence rates of testis cancer in Denmark 1943–96. Points are empirical rates for each combination of age and calendar time in 1-year classes plotted against age. The line represents the predicted incidence rates from a model that specifies log-incidence rates as a linear function of age. The shaded area is the 95% confidence interval for the predicted rates.

CODE EXPLAINED: The `glm` has two explanatory variables (both functions of A), A and A^2. Since the `^` operator has a special meaning in model formulae on the r.h.s. of the ~, the square term must be entered as the argument to the function `I`; for more details see the section on model formulae on p. 74.

The output contains a p-value for the quadratic term, which relates to a test of a null hypothesis of a linear relationship versus that of a quadratic relationship (the alternative)—it is pretty clear that there is strong evidence against the linear relationship with a p-value effectively equal to 0.

The parameters are coefficients of a 2nd degree polynomial, and so not immediately interpretable; the only way we can get a sensible impression of the model is by graphing the predicted values. For the sake of completeness we also graph the predicted rates from the linear model:

```
> pr2 <- ci.pred( m2, newdata=nd )
> matshade( nd$A, cbind(pr2,pr), plot=TRUE )
```

> CODE EXPLAINED: m2 is a `glm` model with two quantitative explanatory variables, A and
> A^2. But since they both are functions of A, the prediction data frame needed to produce
> predicted values from the model is the same as before; we just need values of A to assess
> the contribution from both variables. We can then plot predictions from *both* the linear
> and the quadratic models in the same graph by using `cbind` to put the predictions (with
> confidence limits) from the two models side by side (so that we now have 6 columns).

The figure produced by the code above is not included here.

Further extension to a 3rd degree polynomial is straightforward, but polynomial models
are generally advised against because they occasionally give pretty 'wild' predictions at the
edge of the data:

```
> m3 <- glm( cbind(D,Y/10^5) ~ A + I(A^2) + I(A^3), family=poisreg, data=tdk )
> pr3 <- ci.pred( m3, newdata=nd )
> matshade( nd$A, pr3, plot=TRUE )
```

> CODE EXPLAINED: m3 is a `glm` model with three quantitative explanatory variables, A, A^2,
> and A^3. But since they all are functions of A, the prediction data frame needed to produce
> predicted values from the model is the same as before; we just need values of A to assess
> the contribution from all three variables.
>   We then plot the predictions from the cubic model using `matshade`.

This plot is not shown, because we would like a more elaborate plot, also including the
fits from the linear and quadratic models for comparison:

```
> matshade( nd$A, cbind(pr3,pr2,pr), plot=TRUE,
+           lty=c("solid","32","32"), lend="butt", lwd=2, col=1,
+           log="y", ylim=c(1,20), xlab="Age at FU (years)",
+           ylab="Testis cancer incidence per 100,000 PY" )
```

> CODE EXPLAINED: We plot all 3 predictions from the linear, the quadratic, and the cubic
> models in the same graph by using `cbind` to put the predictions (with confidence limits)
> from the models side by side (so that we now have 9 columns). `matshade` will produce a
> new graph when we set `plot=TRUE`. The type of lines (`lty=`) is a solid line for the cubic
> model and a broken line with three units ink and two units blank ('32') for the linear
> and quadratic models; `lend="butt"` makes the ends of the segments of the broken line
> non-rounded ('butted'). Finally, `log="y"` renders the *y*-axis logarithmic, which is the
> scale on which the estimated effects are linear, quadratic, or cubic.

From Figure 6.2 we see the increasing detail as we add more parameters to the curve,
but also that the 3rd degree polynomial shows a minimum around age 60 and a possible
increase after that. This is an artefact that derives from the mathematical behaviour of a
3rd degree polynomial; it goes from $-\infty$ to $+\infty$ (or vice versa) with a local maximum and
a local minimum in between (well, most do).

Obviously, higher order polynomials can be entertained as well, but these will often
render models that show quite erratic behaviour, so this is not recommended.

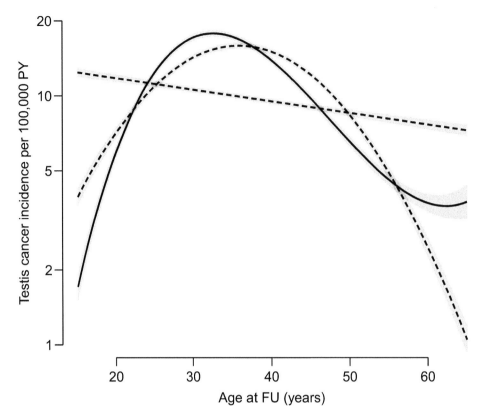

Figure 6.2 Predicted age-specific incidence rates of testis cancer, using linear, quadratic, and cubic model for the age-effect. The cubic effect is shown with a full line; the linear and quadratic effects are shown with broken lines. It is left to the reader to identify which is which.

6.4.4 *Other types of non-linear effects*

More flexible extensions of polynomials for non-linear modelling of effects of quantitative variables exist; the most frequently encountered are fractional polynomials and splines. These methods devise a number of covariates that are functions of the quantitative variable (here A), somewhat more shrewdly thought through than the square and the cube of A, in order to accommodate a smooth non-linear effect of A.

- Fractional polynomials start out with a model with a rich set of power terms (not necessarily integer powers) of the variable and then reduce the model to a smaller set of powers, thus preventing over-fitting. This is an iterative procedure, and is implemented in the mfp package.

  A drawback of fractional polynomial models is that they are not invariant under translation of the variable used, so if you are modelling the effect of calendar time t, say, you will get different models whether you use $t - 1990$ or $t - 2000$ as variable.

  This is the main reason we will not treat fractional polynomials further in this book.

- Splines are models that are piece wise polynomials (normally of degree 1, 2, or 3) between a prespecified set of *knots* and which are required to fit nicely together at the knots. This is done by specifying that the actual values as well as the derivatives must be the same for the two functions joining at each knot. First degree splines are also termed join-point models.

Splines are implemented in the `splines` package (one of the base packages that comes with R) by the functions `bs` and `ns`. The latter is a variant called *natural* splines (or restricted cubic splines), which restricts the function to be linear beyond the first and last defined knots (the boundary knots). The `Ns` function in the `Epi` package is a simplifying wrapper for `ns` that simplifies the specification of knots.

Natural splines with k knots have $k-1$ parameters, and the number of knots is chosen a bit arbitrarily by deciding how many parameters is needed for the effect in question.

Normally the location of the knots is chosen so that the amount of information is approximately the same between each successive pair of knots. It is also possible to use the `gam` function from the `mgcv` package to choose the number and location of knots in an optimal way, using penalized splines.

Natural splines

A very simple application of the `Ns` function shows how the use and prediction from models with splines is quite similar to that from models with simple polynomial terms:

```
> dd <- rep(tdk$A,tdk$D)
> dd <- dd + runif(dd, -0.5, 0.5)
> kk <- quantile(dd, (1:4-0.5)/4 )
> xtabs( D ~ cut(A, c(14,kk,65)), data=tdk )
cut(A, c(14, kk, 65))
  (14,24.1] (24.1,31.1]   (31.1,38]   (38,49.2]   (49.2,65]
       1014        2059        2117        2040        1060
> ms <- glm( cbind(D, Y/10^5) ~ Ns(A, knots=kk), family=poisreg, data=tdk )
> round( ci.lin( ms ), 3 )
                      Estimate StdErr       z     P    2.5%   97.5%
(Intercept)              2.278  0.019 122.462 0.000   2.241   2.314
Ns(A, knots = kk)1      -0.017  0.040  -0.442 0.658  -0.095   0.060
Ns(A, knots = kk)2       0.709  0.039  18.169 0.000   0.633   0.786
Ns(A, knots = kk)3      -0.775  0.029 -26.508 0.000  -0.833  -0.718
```

CODE EXPLAINED: First, we compute positions of the knots so that we have roughly the same number of events between each of the knots; `rep(tdk$A,tdk$D)` creates a vector where each value of `A` in the data frame `tdk` is repeated as many times as `D`, so therefore `dd` is a vector of rounded ages at an event. We add a random noise between −0.5 and 0.5 to mimic the continuous distribution of ages. We then compute the quantiles of these so that approximately 25% are between each pair of knots.

This is shown by `xtabs` that gives the sum of `D` for each level of the factor on the r.h.s., which is a grouping of `A` between the knots (`kk`).

`Ns` generates 3 columns of functions of `A` (one less than the number of knots), so the model uses 3 parameters to describe the age-effect on the incidence rates:

```
> prs <- ci.pred( ms, newdata=nd )
> matshade( nd$A, cbind(prs,pr3,pr2,pr), plot=TRUE,
+           col=gray(c(0,4,4,4)/10),
+           lty=c("solid","32","32","32"), lend="butt",
+           log="y", ylim=c(1,20), lwd=c(4,2,2,2) )
> rug( kk, lwd=2 )
```

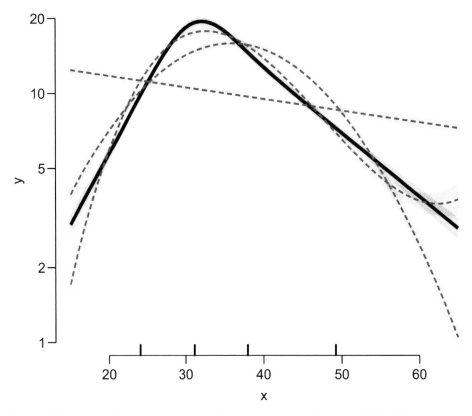

Figure 6.3 Age-specific incidence rates of testis cancer in Denmark (1943–98) using linear, quadratic, cubic, and (natural) spline effects. The broken lines are the 1st, 2nd, and 3rd degree polynomials; the full line is a natural spline with knots indicated by the rug on the x-axis, and so linear beyond the outer knots.

> CODE EXPLAINED: The code for predicting and graphing the rates from this model is precisely the same as for the simple models with quadratic and cubic terms.
>
> rug places marks on the x-axis at the values of the knots. If there were many knots it would look a bit like a carpet—a rug. Hence the name.

From Figure 6.3 we see that the spline model predicts a more pointed peak of incidence rates around age 33 than any of the polynomial fits are able to provide.

Penalized splines

The mgcv package (a package in the standard distribution of R) contains the function gam (generalized additive models) that allows the fitting of models with penalized splines. To cut a long story short, in order to fit a reasonable detailed model without over-fitting data, the gam function fits a model with a large(ish) number of parameters, and in order to prevent the fitted curves from being too wiggly, the curvature (second derivative of the curves—how sharp the bends on the curve are) at any one point needs not to be too large. This is done by contraining the parameters so that the fitted curve meets the curvature requirements. Adding this extra feature to the fitting procedure is called *penalizing* too large curvatures, hence the name penalized splines.

```
> library( mgcv )
> mg <- gam( cbind(D, Y/10^5) ~ s(A, k=15), family=poisreg, data=tdk )
> summary( mg )
Family: poisson
Link function: log

Formula:
cbind(D, Y/10^5) ~ s(A, k = 15)

Parametric coefficients:
            Estimate Std. Error z value Pr(>|z|)
(Intercept)  2.05303    0.01434   143.2   <2e-16

Approximate significance of smooth terms:
       edf Ref.df Chi.sq p-value
s(A) 9.712  11.45   1949  <2e-16

R-sq.(adj) =  0.352   Deviance explained = 37.5%
UBRE = 0.54441  Scale est. = 1        n = 2700
```

> CODE EXPLAINED: The syntax of the gam is similar to that of glm, except for the specification of the covariate effects (the effect of A in this case). The s function specifies a penalized spline, the first argument to s is the covariate, and the k argument is a specification of the maximal number of parameters to use for the modelling.
>
> In this case we used k=15, and the summary shows that the effective number of parameters (edf, effective degrees of freedom) used was 9.7, so the k has not placed any substantial restriction on the modelling; the equivalent of 9–10 parameters was needed for modelling the age-effect.

```
> prg <- ci.pred( mg, newdata=nd )
> matshade( nd$A, cbind( prg, prs ), plot=TRUE,
+           col=1, lwd=2, lty=c("solid","32"), lend="butt",
+           log="y", ylim=c(1,20), xlab="Age",
+           ylab="Testis cancer incidence per 100,000 PY" )
```

> CODE EXPLAINED: The really handy thing is that the prediction machinery is exactly the same as for the glm regardless of what type of smoother is used for the covariate effect, so the matshade function can be used almost unaltered; here we are plotting the fitted curves from the penalized splines (prg) together with those from the model with natural splines (prs).

From Figure 6.4 we see that in this case we get pretty similar results from the two approaches—the penalized spline smooths the curve a bit more. But there is no guarantee that this will always be the case.

Given that the mgcv package is available and provides simple access to smooth functions, it is recommended that the package and the facilities in it be used. The documentation is very detailed, so remember to read it (?gam, ?s).

The main drawback of using the gam modelling in practice may be that it is much slower than the glm, particularly for very large datasets.

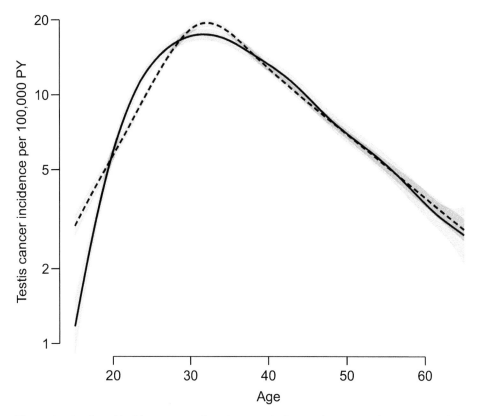

Figure 6.4 Predicted incidence rates of testis cancer in Denmark 1943–96, by age. The solid line is the fit from the penalized spline model (gam); the broken line is from the glm model with a natural spline with 4 knots.

6.5 Two quantitative predictors

The testis cancer incidence data cover a period of almost 50 years, so we would also want to know the shape and size of the effect of calendar time (coded as P). The previous models only tell us about the average rates over the period as a function of age.

6.5.1 *Age and period*

A first step is to include the variable P as a linear effect in the model. Now, if we want to make a prediction of incidence rates from this model we must decide not only on the ages (A) for which we want the prediction but also the dates (P) at which we make the prediction. The gam function also allows the inclusion of a standard linear term in the model:

```
> mgl <- gam( cbind(D,Y/10^5) ~ s(A,k=15) + P, family=poisreg, data=tdk )
> round( ci.lin( mgl, subset="P" ), 4 )

  Estimate StdErr      z P   2.5%  97.5%
P   0.0252  8e-04 33.379 0 0.0237 0.0267

> round( ci.exp( mgl, subset="P" ), 4 )
```

```
      exp(Est.)  2.5%   97.5%
P      1.0255 1.024 1.0271
> nd <- cbind( nd, P=1970 )
> prg1 <- ci.pred( mg1, newdata=nd )
```

CODE EXPLAINED: In the gam function we have just added P in the model, which has the effect of adding a linear effect of calendar time, and which gives an estimate of 0.0252 for P extracted by ci.lin. This means that the incidence rates of testis cancer increase by a factor exp(0.0252) = 1.0255 per year (because this is the units in which P is recorded). So the average annual increase in testis cancer incidence is 2.6%.

We expand the prediction data frame (using cbind) with a column uniformly equal to 1970, so the prediction will refer to incidence rates of testis cancer in 1970. So we can say that the age-specific rates look as if those in the figure increased or decreased by a factor 1.025 per year relative to 1970.

We do not plot the predicted age-specific rates as of 1970—in shape they look pretty much like the overall rates in Figure 6.4.

A natural further step is to see whether there is a non-linear effect of calendar time:

```
> mgp <- gam( cbind(D,Y/10^5) ~ s(A,k=15) + s(P,k=5),
+              family=poisreg, data=tdk )
> summary( mgp )
Family: poisson
Link function: log

Formula:
cbind(D, Y/10^5) ~ s(A, k = 15) + s(P, k = 5)

Parametric coefficients:
            Estimate Std. Error z value Pr(>|z|)
(Intercept)  1.93501    0.01549   124.9   <2e-16

Approximate significance of smooth terms:
       edf Ref.df Chi.sq p-value
s(A) 9.699 11.440   1909  <2e-16
s(P) 2.740  3.252   1086  <2e-16

R-sq.(adj) =  0.595   Deviance explained = 55.7%
UBRE = 0.099507  Scale est. = 1          n = 2700
> anova( mg1, mgp, test="Chisq" )
Analysis of Deviance Table

Model 1: cbind(D, Y/10^5) ~ s(A, k = 15) + P
Model 2: cbind(D, Y/10^5) ~ s(A, k = 15) + s(P, k = 5)
  Resid. Df Resid. Dev    Df Deviance  Pr(>Chi)
1   2686.6     2962.6
2   2684.3     2941.8 2.2491   20.855 4.257e-05
```

CODE EXPLAINED: The gam allows for more non-linear terms; here we set the maximal number of parameters to 5 for the calendar time (P), and the summary reveals that about half of this is needed (the effective degrees of freedom, edf is 2.7).

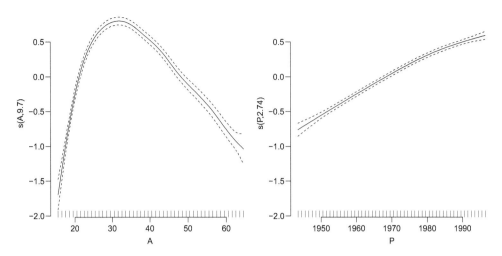

Figure 6.5 Default plot for gam objects with two smooth terms, age (A) and calendar time (P). The 'rugs' at the bottom of each panel are just the positions of the data points.

Like glm, the gam models can be compared using anova, and we see that there is a significant non-linearity by calendar time (P).

We would like to see the effect of calendar time too; a simple and easy plot can be obtained by the default plot method for gam objects:

```
> par( mfrow=c(1,2), mar=c(4,4,0.1,0.1) )
> plot( mgp )
```

CODE EXPLAINED: The par function sets up a layout with two plot frames in a 1×2 layout (mfrow) and sets aside 4 lines of space at the bottom and left, and 0.1 lines of space at the top and right.

The gam object mgp has two smooth terms so the plot function will produce two graphs, one for age (A) and one for calendar time (P); see Figure 6.5.

In this plot, the scales of the y-axes are the log-rate-ratio scale, centred at an overall average. However, we would like to see the graphs of effects that multiplied together give the predicted rates, where the age-effect is interpretable as predicted rates as of 1970, say, and the calendar time effect as the rate ratio relative to this. We already have the first but we need the latter.

While the age-effect is a *prediction* on the scale of the outcome (incidence rates) the calendar time effect we want is a *rate ratio*, a *contrast* relative to some reference point, for example 1970. So for a range of values of P we want the incidence rate ratio between P and 1970. Another way of formulating this is that we want the ratio of two (sets of) predicted incidence rates (those for 1943–98 and those for 1970)—or the difference between two log-predictions and the transform of these to rate ratios.

There is a machinery for this in the Epi package; if a list of two prediction frames is supplied to ci.exp (or ci.lin) as the argument ctr.mat, it will return the ratio of the predictions with confidence intervals:

```
> par( mfrow=c(1,2) )
> matshade( nd$A, ci.pred( mgp, nd ), plot=TRUE,
+           log="y",  ylim=c(1,20), xlim=13+c(0,53),
+           xlab="Age", ylab="Testis cancer incidence 1970 (per 100,00 PY)" )
> np <- data.frame( A=30, P=1943:1996 )
> nr <- data.frame( A=30, P=1970 )
> RR <- ci.exp( mgp, ctr.mat=list(np,nr) )
> matshade( np$P, RR, plot=TRUE,
+           log="y",  ylim=c(1,20)/4, xlim=1943+c(0,53),
+           xlab="Date of FU", ylab="Incidence RR relative to 1970" )
> abline( h=1, v=1970, lty=3 )
```

CODE EXPLAINED: As before, we set up two panels side by side, and plot the predicted age-specific rates as of 1970 in the first with proper axis notation (using xlab and ylab), and with length of the *x*-axis 53 years, and the extent of the *y*-axis (which is logarithmic) 1:20.

For the RRs we construct two prediction data frames, one (np) for the numerator, and one (nr) for the denominator—the reference. Either the two data frames should have the same number of rows or the second should have only one row; in the latter case the row will be replicated to match the number of rows in the first. ci.exp returns a rate ratio with c.i. for each row of the prediction frame np. We used A=30 in the prediction frames, but the model is a main-effects model so the rate ratios would be the same in any age.

We plot the RR on a log-scale, and explicitly scale the axes to be as in the first plot, the *x*-axis 53 years long and the *y*-axis with a ratio 20 between the upper and lower end (because it is a logarithmic axis). This way the two effects will be comparable. The specification of the *y*-axis in the RR plot is via an arithmetic expression (ylim=c(1,20)/4), which makes it clear that the relative extent is the same as for the age-effect; using ylim=c(0.25,5) would obscure this. This shows one major advantage of R: you can always use an arithmetic expression instead of a vector or the name of a variable; in this case we used the feature to make the common scaling of *y*-axes clear in the code.

Note that the data are grouped in 1-year intervals, but since we have coded age and calendar time as quantitative variables (by the midpoint of the intervals) and use them as such, the reference for calendar time is not a period such as the year of 1970, but a specific date. We used the value P=1970 which corresponds to 1 January 1970.

Inspection of the plot from this piece of code would reveal a classical problem with multiple plots in R: too much white space around the plots. This is, however, fairly easily fixed, by shrinking the margin space and correspondingly the placement of the axis titles and annotation by using the following:

```
> par( mfrow=c(1,2), mar=c(3,3,0.1,0.1), mgp=c(3,1,0)/1.6 )
> matshade( nd$A, ci.pred( mgp, nd ), plot=TRUE,
+           log="y", ylim=c(1,20), xlim=13+c(0,53),
+           xlab="Age at FU",
+           ylab="Testis cancer incidence 1970 (per 100,00 PY)" )
> np <- data.frame( A=30, P=1943:1996 )
> nr <- data.frame( A=30, P=1970 )
> RR <- ci.exp( mgp, ctr.mat=list(np,nr) )
> matshade( np$P, RR, plot=TRUE,
```

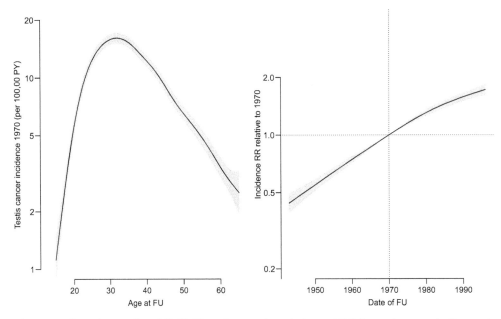

Figure 6.6 Rates by age for 1970-01-01, and rate ratios relative to 1970 for testis cancer in Denmark 1943–1996 in ages 15–65. Estimates are from a gam model with main effects of age and calendar time. We see a 10-fold increase in rates from age 15 to 30, and a 5-fold decrease from age 30 to 65, and a steady increase by calendar time, tending to level off in the later years.

```
+               log="y",  ylim=c(1,20)/5,  xlim=1943+c(0,53),
+               xlab="Date of FU", ylab="Incidence RR relative to 1970" )
> abline( h=1, v=1970, lty=3 )
```

> CODE EXPLAINED: We have changed the mar argument in the par function, so that we only have 3 (and not 4) lines of space at the bottom and left. The default placement of axis titles is at line 3, and numbering at line 1, so this must be changed. These are governed by the argument mgp which has a default of c(3,1,0), so we shrink this by a factor 1.6. The rest is the same as above; the result is in Figure 6.6.

6.5.2 *Age and cohort*

For the sake of completeness we may consider date of birth (occasionally termed 'cohort') instead of date of follow-up as the second quantitative variable; so we form this variable:

```
> tdk$B <- tdk$P - tdk$A
> range( tdk$B )
[1] 1879 1981
```

When modelling incidence rates by age and date of birth, the age-effect will be what is normally called a *longitudinal* age-effect; it will refer to how the age-specific incidence rates evolve for a group of persons born at a given time. Such a group of persons is normally referred to as a birth cohort, hence the name 'cohort' for the variable 'date of birth'.

The simplest possible model is one with a linear effect of date of birth (B); however, this is the same as the model with a linear effect of P:

```
> mlc <- gam( cbind(D,Y/10^5) ~ s(A,k=15) + B, family=poisreg, data=tdk )
> mlp <- gam( cbind(D,Y/10^5) ~ s(A,k=15) + P, family=poisreg, data=tdk )
> rbind( ci.exp(mlc,subset="B"),
+        ci.exp(mlp,subset="P") )
  exp(Est.)      2.5%     97.5%
B  1.025532 1.024015 1.027051
P  1.025532 1.024015 1.027051
> library( dplyr )
> table( fitted(mlc)==fitted(mlp) )
FALSE   TRUE
 2516    184
> table( near( fitted(mlc), fitted(mlp) ) )
TRUE
2700
```

> CODE EXPLAINED: We use `ci.exp` to extract the linear parameter for B, respectively P, from each of the models, and stack them by `rbind` to demonstrate that they are the same.
>
> If we try to see whether the fitted values from the two models are identical by using '`==`' we find that they are not; only a small fraction are. This is the ubiquitous problem of the inaccurate representation of numbers in a computer. So never ask whether numbers are identical; ask whether they are very close. For this purpose we use the function `near` from `dplyr` to assess whether the fitted values from the two models are close. `near` returns a logical vector, and we see that all values are TRUE, so the two models *do* yield the same fitted values—bar estimation inaccuracy.

The two models are identical because $b = p - a$, so an age-effect plus a linear term in period, p, can be written as a different age-effect plus a linear term in b:

$$f(a) + \gamma p = f(a) + \gamma p - \gamma a + \gamma a = f(a) + \gamma(p - a) + \gamma a = (f(a) + \gamma a) + \gamma b$$

The fitted rates will be the same, but the age-effect will be different in the two models.

Fitting the model with a non-linear cohort effect instead of a non-linear period effect produces a different model, but the code is very similar:

```
> mgc <- gam( cbind(D,Y/10^5) ~ s(A,k=15) + s(B,k=40),
+             family=poisreg, data=tdk )
> summary( mgc )
Family: poisson
Link function: log

Formula:
cbind(D, Y/10^5) ~ s(A, k = 15) + s(B, k = 40)

Parametric coefficients:
            Estimate Std. Error z value Pr(>|z|)
(Intercept)  1.95030    0.01567   124.5   <2e-16

Approximate significance of smooth terms:
        edf Ref.df Chi.sq p-value
s(A)  9.708  11.45   1388  <2e-16
s(B) 11.278  14.11   1188  <2e-16
```

```
R-sq.(adj) =  0.604    Deviance explained = 56.3%
UBRE = 0.08951  Scale est. = 1         n = 2700

> anova( mgp, mgl, mgc, test="Chisq" )
Analysis of Deviance Table

Model 1: cbind(D, Y/10^5) ~ s(A, k = 15) + s(P, k = 5)
Model 2: cbind(D, Y/10^5) ~ s(A, k = 15) + P
Model 3: cbind(D, Y/10^5) ~ s(A, k = 15) + s(B, k = 40)
  Resid. Df Resid. Dev      Df Deviance  Pr(>Chi)
1    2684.3     2941.8
2    2686.6     2962.6 -2.2491  -20.855 4.257e-05
3    2673.4     2897.7 13.1212   64.940 7.502e-09

> c( mgp$aic, mgl$aic, mgc$aic )
[1] 9422.079 9439.459 9395.085
```

> CODE EXPLAINED: The model with date of birth (B) is fitted exactly as the model with the date of follow-up (P), except we allow for 40 parameters for the B in order to accommodate potential short-term fluctuations of the effects.
>   The anova compares the model with the linear effect of P (mgl) with both the extensions—note that the model with a single linear term is in the middle.
>   We use the $aic to extract the AIC from the model objects.

The deviance difference is substantially larger for the cohort model (64.9 vs 20.9), meaning that the (non-linear part of) cohort accounts for more of the variation in data than the non-linear part for the period. On the other hand, the cohort model also has more parameters (the d.f. differences are 11.3 vs 2.7), but we also see that the AIC is substantially smaller for the cohort model.

When we plot the age and cohort effects we should recognize that the agerange is about 50 years, but that date of birth spans some 100 years, so we use the layout to produce plot panels of different widths:

```
> par( mar=c(3,3,0.1,0.1), mgp=c(3,1,0)/1.6 )
> layout( rbind(1:2), widths=c(1,1.8) )
> na   <- data.frame( A=15:65, B=1930 )
> matshade( na$A, ci.pred( mgc, na ), plot=TRUE,
+           log="y",  ylim=c(1,20), xlim=13+c(0,53), xlab="Age at FU",
+           ylab="Testis cancer incidence: 1930 cohort (per 100,000 PY)" )
> nc   <- data.frame( A=30, B=1880:1980 )
> ncr <- data.frame( A=30, B=1930 )
> RRc <- ci.exp( mgc, ctr.mat=list(nc,ncr) )
> matshade( nc$B, RRc, plot=TRUE,
+           log="y",  ylim=c(1,20)/5, xlim=1878+c(0,106),
+           xlab="Date of birth", ylab="Incidence RR relative to 1930
          cohort" )
> abline( h=1, v=c(1930,1918+10/12,1945+5/12), lty=3 )
```

> CODE EXPLAINED: The prediction data frame for the cohort effect (nc) has a range of 100 years, so in order to get the slopes comparable between age and cohort we use layout to devise a plot with two panels where the second is wider (the widths argument)—a bit of trial and error was exercised to attain approximately the same physical extent of 10 years on the x-axis in both panels (Figure 6.7). The rest of the derivation and plotting of predicted rates and RRs is exactly as for the model with P.

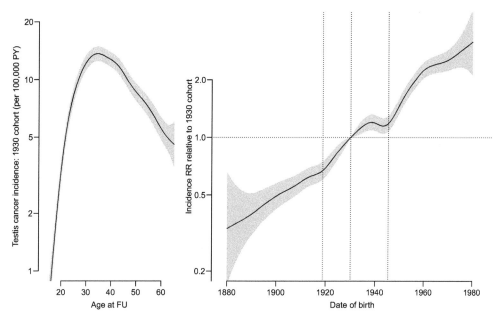

Figure 6.7 Rates by age for men born 1930-01-01, and rate ratios relative to this for testis cancer in Denmark 1943–1996 in ages 15–65. Estimates are from a `gam` model with main effects of age and date of birth.

In the cohort plot (Figure 6.7, right) is a vertical line (`abline` argument v) at the reference cohort (1930), but also at the end of WW1 (October 1918) and WW2 (May 1945) to show the effect of the wars on the birth cohorts' future incidence of testis cancer.

6.5.3 *Contours of joint effects*

In order to visualize the rates as modelled by age and period we can estimate the rates in a grid from 15 to 65 years of age and from dates 1943 through 1998, that is, 50 by 55 years:

```
> nd <- expand.grid( A=15:65, P=1943:1998 )
> nd$B <- nd$P-nd$A
> nd$Prate <- ci.pred( mgp, nd )[,1]
> nd$Brate <- ci.pred( mgc, nd )[,1]
> head( nd, 4 )
   A    P    B     Prate      Brate
1 15 1943 1928 0.4931584 0.5717171
2 16 1943 1927 0.7006321 0.8040160
3 17 1943 1926 0.9905546 1.1234755
4 18 1943 1925 1.3788471 1.5430942
```

CODE EXPLAINED: `expand.grid` generates a data frame with one record per combination of age (A) and calendar time (P) of follow-up; from these we generate the dates of birth (B) by subtracting age (A) from current date (P). For each record of this data frame we generate the predicted rates from the two models we fitted with age and respectively period and cohort effects, omitting the confidence intervals using '`[,1]`' to fish out only the first column with the predicted rates.

With the predicted rates from the two models in the nd data frame we can now use ggplot to draw contour plots:

```
> library( ggplot2 )
> library( gridExtra )
> library( ggthemes )
> cp <- ggplot( nd, aes(P, A, z=log(Prate)) ) +
+               geom_contour( binwidth = log(1.5), col=1 ) +
+               theme_tufte( base_size = 24,
+                            base_family = "Helvetica" )
> cb <- ggplot( nd, aes(P, A, z=log(Brate)) ) +
+               geom_contour( binwidth = log(1.5), col=1 ) +
+               theme_tufte( base_size = 24,
+                            base_family = "Helvetica" ) +
+               geom_abline( intercept = -c(1945+5/12,1918+10/12),
+                            slope = 1,
+                            color = gray(0.4) ) +
+               geom_label( aes(label=c("1918","1945")),
+                           data=data.frame(P = c(1983,1998),
+                                           A = c(  65,   53),
+                                           Brate = NA) )
> grid.arrange(cp, cb, nrow=1)
```

CODE EXPLAINED: We use the generated dataset nd and from that the log-rates as z-variable (z=log(Prate)). The reason for using the log rates is that we want contour lines to represent successive levels of rates at a given *relative* distance; using binwidth=log(1.5) in geom_contour we obtain that successive contours represent (estimated) rates that differ by 50% (a rate ratio of 1.5).

The theme_tufte minimizes the amount of chart-junk and renders the graph nice and clean, according to Tufte's principles.[1] The font size (base_size) was determined by trial and error.

To illustrate the characteristic dip in the effect of date of birth around the end of WW1 and WW2, we used geom_abline in the second graph to put in two lines indicating these two cohorts. In order to put labels on the two cohort lines we use geom_label where the points where the labels go are given in a data frame supplied in a data argument.

Note that we assigned the plots to so-called grobs (graphical objects), cp and cb, so no graphs are actually plotted by the ggplot statements. The graphs are plotted side by side by the grid.arrange function asking for the graphs to be displayed in a single row (nrow=1).

As opposed to the plots in Figures 6.6 and 6.7, the contour plots in Figure 6.8 do not allow the uncertainty of rates in terms of confidence intervals to be incorporated. Also it is not immediately discernible from the contour plots how the two components contribute to the estimated rates.

Image plot / heatmap

In general, contour plots are difficult to read; images (or heatmaps as they are also called) are a bit easier to read because they colour the age–period area according to the size of the

---

[1] Edward Tufte, *The Visual Display of Quantitative Information*, Graphics Press (1983).

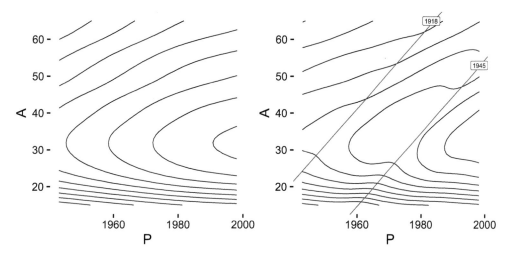

Figure 6.8 Contour plots of the estimated rates of testis cancer in Denmark. (Left) The estimated rates from the gam model with main effects of age and date of FU. (Right) The gam model with main effects of age and date of birth. Successive contours represent rates with a ratio of 1.5.

rates. You can think of a heatmap as a colouring of the areas between the contours of a contour plot. Or as a good old-fashioned school map showing mountains and valleys.

The base graphics function image does the trick, but we first need a few things to pass on to the image function; a matrix of values for a grid of points by age and period, as well as the vectors of the classifying ages and periods:

```
> lrP <- xtabs( log(Prate) ~ P + A, data=nd )
> lrB <- xtabs( log(Brate) ~ P + A, data=nd )
> Age    <- as.numeric( colnames(lrP) )
> Period <- as.numeric( rownames(lrP) )
> rng <- range( c(log(nd$Prate),
+                    log(nd$Brate)) )
> brk <- seq( rng[1], rng[2], length=13 )
> exp( diff(brk)[1] )
[1] 1.418162
```

CODE EXPLAINED: image requires a matrix (or table) as input, so we use xtabs to generate a matrix of the log-predicted rates. image will plot rows of the matrix in columns on the plot, somewhat illogical. So we make P the rowvariable by putting it first in xtabs. xtabs produces a table with the *sum* of the l.h.s. variable, within each combination of the r.h.s. variables; but the way nd were generated there is only one record for each combination of P and A, so xtabs is merely used as a machinery to arrange data in a matrix.

We will also need the numerical values of age and period that classified the matrix, so we derive these from the matrix lrP; note that we called the period and age values Period and Age, since this will be the axis labels by default.

Finally, image needs an argument breaks that determine what intervals of the response variable (log rates, in this case) gets each colour. We take these as 13 equidistant values over the range of the log rates—one more than the number of colours which by default is 12.

rng is the range of all fitted log-rate values for the two models, and seq generates 13 equidistant numbers from the smallest (rng[1]) to the largest (rng[2]).

The difference between elements of brk is the log-RR between successive groups; we see it corresponds to a RR of about 1.4.

```
> par( mfrow=c(1,2), mar=c(3,3,0.1,0.1), mgp=c(3,1,0)/1.6 )
> image( x  =Period, y = Age, z = lrP, breaks=brk )
> text( 1945, 64, "Age-period model", adj=0 )
> image( x = Period, y = Age, z = lrB, breaks=brk )
> text( 1945, 64, "Age-cohort model", adj=0 )
> abline(-1945,1)
> abline(-1918,1)
> text( 1995, 1995-1945.2, "1945", adj=c(1,0) )
> text( 1975, 1975-1918.2, "1918", adj=c(1,0) )
```

CODE EXPLAINED: We then set up a plot with two panels using mfrow= and produce image plots for the fitted values from the period, respectively cohort model. The first argument (x) is the columndimension of the z argument; the second argument (y) is the rowdimension of z. The final plot will be with x on the horizontal axis and y on the vertical axis.

The brk has 13 values, corresponding to 12 intervals of separate colour for the (log-) rates—the default is 12 colours, but this can also be changed; try ?image.

The abline draws a line with a given intercept and slope; an intercept (crossing the y-axis) of −1945 and a slope of 1 means that the line crosses the x-axis at 1945; hence, it represents the 1945 birth-cohort. Finally, text puts labels on the two cohortlines.

In the left panel of Figure 6.9 we see the increase of rates along the x-axis, the age–period model asserts that the age-effect has the same shape at any given age, so the peak is

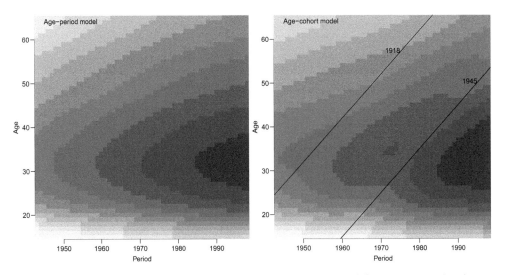

Figure 6.9 Image plots of the estimated rates of testis cancer in Denmark from age–period and age–cohort models. (Left) The estimated rates from the gam model with the main effects of age and date of follow-up. (Right) The gam model with the main effects of age and date of birth. The relative span of rates within each colour is approximately 1.4.

necessarily at the same age ($\approx$ 32) at any date. In the right panel the age-effects along the diagonals indicated have the same shape but vary by the birth cohort. We can just see a little increase of the peak in a cohort a few years before the 1945 cohort.

6.6 Quantitative interactions

6.6.1 *Age–period interaction*

In our data example we have two quantitative variables: age and calendar time (as well as their difference, date of birth). The model we fitted in the previous section were *main effects* models, where the effect of age (A) was assumed to be the same across all dates (P) and vice versa. A possible extension of the model would be one where the age-effects were assumed to vary by date. One possible way of doing this is to use the capability in gam to fit models with a two-dimensional spline function:

```
> miap <- gam( cbind(D,Y/10^5) ~ s(A,P,k=50), family=poisreg, data=tdk )
> anova( mgp, miap, mgc, test="Chisq" )
Analysis of Deviance Table

Model 1: cbind(D, Y/10^5) ~ s(A, k = 15) + s(P, k = 5)
Model 2: cbind(D, Y/10^5) ~ s(A, P, k = 50)
Model 3: cbind(D, Y/10^5) ~ s(A, k = 15) + s(B, k = 40)
  Resid. Df Resid. Dev      Df Deviance  Pr(>Chi)
1    2684.3    2941.8
2    2654.3    2829.5  29.986   112.25 1.954e-11
3    2673.4    2897.7 -19.114   -68.16 2.005e-07

> c( ap=mgp$aic, api=miap$aic, ac=mgc$aic )
      ap       api        ac
9422.079 9360.989 9395.085
```

> CODE EXPLAINED: The s function allows for more than one variable, so the specification of both A and P as arguments fits an interaction model. The anova compares the model with period effect (mgp), the interaction model miap, and the model with cohort effect (mgc).
> Even though the age–cohort model is not formally a submodel of the age–period interaction model we compare the deviance of this to the interaction model.
> We also compare the models using AIC, extracted directly from the models.

We see that the distance between the interaction model and the age–period model in terms of deviance (Deviance in the anova output) is larger than that between the interaction model and the age–cohort model. This is also seen from the values of the AICs.

However, once we have established that there is some sort of interaction between A and P, it remains to show *how* the interaction looks.

Reporting the effects in a model with interaction between quantitative variables can in principle be done in a 3-dimensional plot where the predicted rates are shown as a response surface over an age-by-period grid, or we could use either a contour plot or a heatmap. But for these types of plot it is not possible to include confidence limits of the predictions, and despite the fancy looks they are difficult to interpret.

Age-specific rates at different dates (periods)

It is easier to understand the shape of the interaction if we plot several age-specific incidence curves together, each representing the age-specific rates at a given period—this corresponds to cuts in the surface at a set of dates in the age direction. So the basic idea is to choose a limited number of dates for which we will predict the age-specific rates, and then plot these together:

```
> yr <- seq(1950, 1990, 8)
> cl <- gray( seq(0.7, 0.1, length=6) )
> np <- data.frame( A=seq(15,65,0.5) )
> plot( NA, log="y", ylim=c(0.5,30), xlim=c(15,65),
+           xlab="Age at FU", ylab="Incidence rate per 100,000 PY" )
> for( i in 1:length(yr) )
+     {
+ np$P <- yr[i] ; np$B <- np$P-np$A
+ matshade( np$A, ci.pred(miap,np), col=cl[i] )
+     }
> text(65,30*0.85^(5:0),yr,adj=1,col=cl)
> wh.a <- c(30:32,31:33)
> text(wh.a,ci.pred(miap,data.frame(A=wh.a,P=yr))[,1],yr,cex=0.6)
```

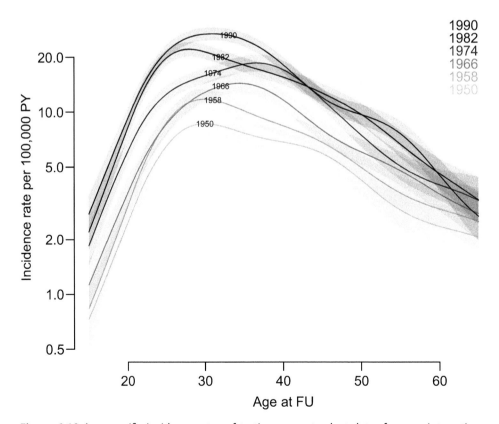

Figure 6.10 Age-specific incidence rates of testis cancer at select dates from an interaction model. Each curve represents the (predicted) age-specific incidence rates at a given date.

CODE EXPLAINED: The vector yr holds the dates at which we will plot the rates as a function of age, and cl is given the colours we will use for the curves, in this case grey tones between 0.8 (light) and 0.1 (dark). nd is the prediction data frame for ages between 15 and 65, and we intend to expand it by yr.

The plot function with first argument NA plots an empty graph; xlim specifies the extent of the x-axis, ylim the extent of the y-axis, while log="y" requires that the y-axis is logarithmic, and xlab and ylab specify the annotation of the two axes.

The for loop has an index i running from 1 to length(yr)—the dates are fished out of yr using i and inserted in the prediction data frame nd as the variable P (as a constant in the data frame). This updated data frame np is used to derive a prediction from the model by ci.pred for all ages and one fixed date, which is plotted with c.i. using matshade—matshade by default just adds a line with shaded confidence interval. The colours for the lines by the matshade function are also found using the loop-variable i as cl[i].

As legend, the dates at which the predictions are computed are written in the colours of the corresponding curves in the top right corner. Note that since the y-axis is logarithmic, the spacing of the vertical position is multiplicative; we multiply the top vertical position, 50, successively by 0.85 for the position of the legends.

For illustration we also put the dates on the curves; by visual inspection of the curves we decided the x values (ages) at which the curves should be annotated (in wh.a), and then used ci.pred to compute the corresponding values on the curves. Note that wh.a both appear as x-coordinate in text (the first argument), and as component of the prediction data frame in ci.pred. This is the way to plot the dates on top of the correct lines.

We see that there is a good reason that the model with main effect of age (A) and date (P) provides such a poor fit; if that model were the true model the curves in Figure 6.10 would be parallel, which they are certainly not. It appears that early increases (1950–70) have been in ages over 30, whereas later increases have mainly been in younger ages.

The annotation of the curves is used to illustrate that standard legends may be improved by putting the annotation directly in the graph; usually this is best done by using text. Moreover, note that since the curves are *ordered* by date, the colouring of the curves should reflect the ordering either as here by grey tones or by some set of colours. An arbitrary set of colours should be avoided when ordered curves (or points) are plotted.

Period-specific rates at different ages

We could also have chosen to show the time-course of the incidence rates at select ages, so to speak slicing the surface at a set of ages in the calendar time direction; this would basically just be interchanging the roles of A and P:

```
> ag <- seq(15,65,10)
> cl <- gray(seq(.6,.1,length=6))
> np <- data.frame( P=seq(1945,1995,0.5) )
> plot( NA, log="y", ylim=c(0.5,30), xlim=c(1945,1995),
+          xlab="Date of FU", ylab="Incidence rate per 100,000 PY" )
> for( i in 1:6 )
+    {
+ np$A <- ag[i]
+ matshade( np$P, ci.pred(miap,np), col=cl[i] )
+    }
> text(1945,30*0.85^(5:0),ag,adj=0,col=cl)
```

```
> wh.p <- 1984
> text( wh.p, ci.pred( miap, data.frame(A=ag,P=wh.p) )[,1],
+       ag, cex=0.6 )
```

CODE EXPLAINED: This code is derived from the previous, but now with 6 ages (in ag) instead of 6 dates, and a curve along time from 1945 through 1995 (in the prediction data frame nd), instead of along ages. The resulting figure is 6.11.

The main effects would also imply that the curves in Figure 6.11 would be parallel, but they are not. If anything it seems that the younger age classes have a steeper slope by calendar time than the older ages.

The practical reporting (description) of the shape of the interaction is not a trivial task from neither Figure 6.11 or Figure 6.11. In many practical cases we might find a significant interaction, but no usable way of describing it. The two plots devised here should be made whenever a quantitative-by-quantitative interaction model is used. Finally, it is pretty clear that annotating of curves directly *on* the curves makes it much easier to distinguish which is which, although it take a little effort to do so.

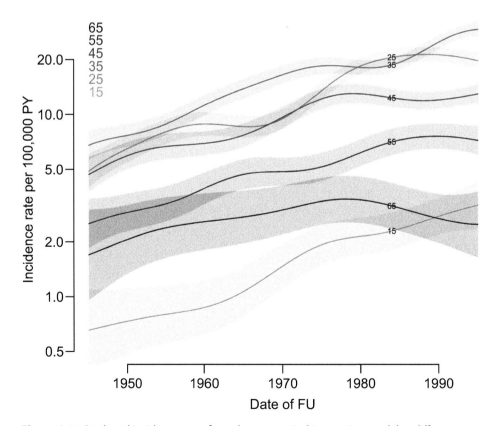

Figure 6.11 Predicted incidence rates from the age–period interaction model at different ages as functions of calendar time. Each curve represents the (predicted) incidence rates at a given age as a function of calendar time.

6.6.2 *Age and cohort interaction*

This section is very code-intensive, and can easily be skipped. It is intended to illustrate the same concepts in a more complicated situation—unlike age and period, not all values of age appear for all dates of birth and vice versa.

As for the main effects models, we can also substitute P with B (date of birth) for the interaction model. This would be an extension of the model where the age-effects were assumed to vary by date of birth. One possible way of doing this is as before to use the capability in gam to fit models with a two-dimensional spline function.

The entire exercise with the age–cohort interaction is parallel to that for the age–period interaction with the exception that plotting curves becomes a bit more complicated from the fact that the birth cohorts are observed in different age spans.

```
> miac <- gam( cbind(D,Y/10^5) ~ s(A,B,k=60), family=poisreg, data=tdk )
> anova( mgp, miac, mgc, test="Chisq" )
Analysis of Deviance Table

Model 1: cbind(D, Y/10^5) ~ s(A, k = 15) + s(P, k = 5)
Model 2: cbind(D, Y/10^5) ~ s(A, B, k = 60)
Model 3: cbind(D, Y/10^5) ~ s(A, k = 15) + s(B, k = 40)
  Resid. Df Resid. Dev     Df Deviance   Pr(>Chi)
1    2684.3    2941.8
2    2645.5    2815.6  38.846  126.201  3.626e-11
3    2673.4    2897.7 -27.974  -82.115  3.170e-07

> c( ap=mgp$aic, iap=miap$aic, iac=miac$aic, ac=mgc$aic )
      ap       iap       iac        ac
9422.079 9360.989 9362.036 9395.085
```

> CODE EXPLAINED: The s function allows for more than one variable, so the specification of both A and B as arguments fits an interaction model. The anova compares the model with period effect (mgp), the interaction models miap and miac, and the model with cohort effect (mgc).
>
> We also compare the models using AIC, extracted directly from the model objects. Note we also included the AIC from the previous age-by-period interaction model.

From a formal point of view, the interaction models are clearly superior to any of the main-effects models, but the difference in AIC between the two interaction models is very small relative to the differences to the main effects models.

Similar to what was done with the age–period interaction we can show the age-specific rates for select dates of birth, or the birth-date-specific rates for select ages. We start with the former:

```
> bc <- seq(1900,1970,10)
> cl <- gray(seq(0.7,0.1,length=8))
> plot( NA, log="y", ylim=c(0.5,30), xlim=c(15,65),
+         xlab="Age at FU", ylab="Incidence rate per 100,000 PY" )
> for( i in 1:8 )
+   {
+ nc <- subset( data.frame( A=seq(15,65,0.5), B=bc[i] ),
+                 A+B>1943 & A+B<1998 )
+ nc$P <- nc$A + nc$B
```

```
+ matshade( nc$A, ci.pred(miac,nc), col=cl[i] )
+ matshade( nc$A, ci.pred(miap,nc), col=cl[i],
+            alpha=0, lty="44", lend="butt" )
+    }
> text(65,30,"Date of birth",adj=1)
> text(65,30*0.85^(8:1),bc,adj=1,col=cl)
```

CODE EXPLAINED: The vector bc is given the birth dates for which we will plot the age-specific rates, and cl is given the colours we will use for the curves, in this case 8 grey tones between 0.7 (light) and 0.1 (dark). nd is the prediction data frame for ages between 15 and 65, and the first birth date in bc. However, not all ages are represented for all birth dates in the original data, so in order to avoid predictions outside of the actual data we restrict the prediction data frame to the follow-up from 1943 through 1998—the date of follow-up is A+B.

Then we make an empty plot (by plotting NA), and specify the x and y limits and axis titles.

The for loop has an index i running from 1 to 8—the date of birth is fished out of bc using this and inserted in the prediction data frame nd, which is then subsetted to the period range 1943–96. Note that the subsetting exercise is *inside* the loop, because each birth cohort has a different age-span of follow-up. The remaining colours for the lines inside the matshade function are also found using the loop-variable i. For comparison we plot the predictions both for the age–cohort (miac) and for the age–period (miap) interaction models. The confidence intervals from the miap model are suppressed by setting the transparency parameter alpha to 0, which means completely transparent (invisible).

As legend, the dates at which the predictions are computed are written in the colours of the corresponding curves in the top right corner. Note that since the y-axis is logarithmic, the spacing of the vertical position is multiplicative; we multiply the top vertical position (30) successively by 0.85.

If the main-effects model with effects of A and B were adequate, the interaction model would produce essentially parallel curves in Figure 6.12, which is not so far off the mark as suggested by the AICs for the models. Also we see that the fitted rates from the age–period and the age–cohort interaction models are quite similar, not surprising, because both are models that fit a flexible model for combinations of age and period.

We can also show the incidence rates at select ages in different birth cohorts, so to speak slicing the surface at a set of ages in the birth date direction—this would basically just be interchanging the roles of A and B:

```
> ag <- seq(15,65,10)
> cl <- gray(seq(.7,.1,length=6))
> plot( NA, log="y", ylim=c(0.5,30), xlim=c(1880,1980),
+        xlab="Date of birth", ylab="Incidence rate per 100,000 PY" )
> for( i in 1:6 )
+    {
+ nb <- subset( data.frame( B=1880:1980, A=ag[i] ),
+               A+B>1943 & A+B<1998 )
+ matshade( nb$B, ci.pred(miac,nb), col=cl[i] )
+    }
> text(1880,30,"Age",adj=0)
> text(1880,30*0.85^(6:1),ag,adj=0,col=cl)
```

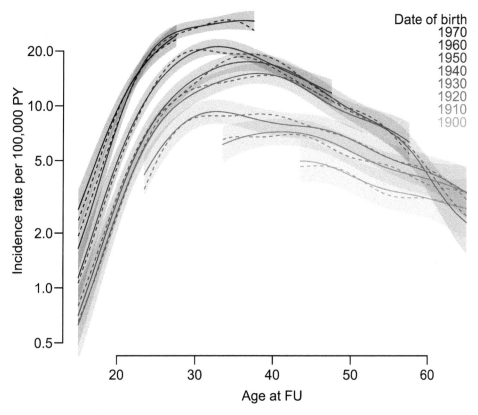

Figure 6.12 Age-specific testis cancer incidence rates from models with interaction between age and period/cohort. Full curves are from the age–cohort interaction model; broken curves are from the age–period interaction model. The shaded areas are 95% confidence intervals.

```
> wh.p <- 1988
> text( wh.p-ag,
+        ci.pred(miac,data.frame(A=ag,B=wh.p-ag))[,1],
+        ag, cex=0.6 )
```

CODE EXPLAINED: This code is derived from the previous, but now with 6 ages (in ag) instead of 8 dates, and a curve along birth date from 1880 through 1980 (or the part of it for which we actually have data).

Note that we use the dates of follow-up wh.p for annotation and translate to the relevant birth cohort by subtracting the age (ag).

A main-effects model with age and cohort would imply that the curves in Figure 6.11 would be parallel, but they are clearly not; it seems that the younger age classes have a steeper slope by calendar time than the older ages.

The practical reporting (description) of the shape of the interaction is not a trivial task neither from Figure 6.12 or Figure 6.13. In many practical cases we might find a significant interaction, but no usable way of describing it. The two types of line plots devised here should be made whenever a quantitative-by-quantitative interaction model is used. One important reason is that these plots allows confidence intervals to help guide the interpretation of the curves.

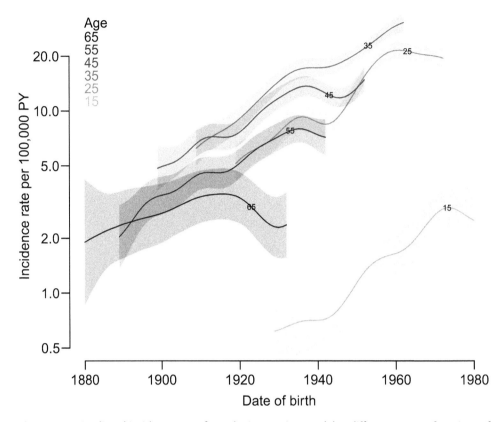

Figure 6.13 Predicted incidence rates from the interaction model at different ages as functions of date of birth.

6.6.3 *Parametric interaction models*

The interaction models we considered were based on two-dimensional splines implemented in the s function in the mgcv package. It is, however, possible to specify more restrictive interactions between quantitative variables.

The very simplest is just to include the product of the two quantitative variables in the model; it will give an indication of whether the interaction is tantamount to a joint effect of both—some call it synergy. This can be viewed as a first step towards fractional polynomials (see p. 130) for the product.

Another variant is to include the sum or the difference between the two variables. A particular case of this is the age–period–cohort models where non-linear functions of age, period, and cohort are used. These can be seen as an extension of the age–period model with a non-linear term of the difference between period and age, the cohort. But they can also be seen as an extension of the age–cohort model with a non-linear term of the sum of age and cohort, the period.

The age–period–cohort model is over-parametrized because it both contains age and period as well as the difference between the two. This has caused a lot of confusion in the literature, with many resulting fallacies, most prominently the Boyle–Robertson fallacy [8]. The details of this topic is beyond this book, but an overview in the vein of this chapter can be found in my article about such models [3].

6.6.4 Varying coefficients models for interaction

Another restricted approach to the interaction instead of a completely unspecified function of the variables A and P is the *varying coefficients* model.

The models we explored in the previous section can be written

$$\log\left(\lambda(a,p)\right) = f(a) + g(p), \qquad \log\left(\lambda(a,p)\right) = f(a,p)$$

If we want to explore whether the time trend is different across ages we may specify what is called a time-varying coefficients model for the interaction:

$$\log\left(\lambda(a,p)\right) = f(a) + g(p) + \gamma(a)p$$

Here the interaction is a product of a smooth function of a and a linear term in p. This has the consequence that if we look at the difference in time trends between two ages, say age a relative to some reference age, a_0, we will have

$$\log\left(\lambda(a,p)\right) - \log\left(\lambda(a_0,p)\right) = \left(f(a) - f(a_0)\right) + \left(\gamma(a) - \gamma(a_0)\right)p = \alpha_a + \beta_a p$$

This means that we have constrained the calendar time trends in rates at different ages to differ only by a linear term in calendar time, so a more restrictive form of interaction. One way of reporting this would be to show the lines $\alpha_a + \beta_a p$ relative to the horizontal line for the reference age for select values of a. However, this will add little to a display of the estimated calendar time trends for select values of a, $\log(\lambda_a(p)) = f(a) + g(p) + \gamma(a)p$.

Note that this extension of the main-effects model is *a*symmetric; another possible extension of the main-effects model introduces an extra linear effect of age:

$$\log\left(\lambda(a,p)\right) = f(a) + g(p) + \xi(p)a$$

It is a subject-matter decision as to which one to use, but both are extensions of the age–period model, and both are submodels of the age-by-period interaction model.

In some applications the varying coefficients model is defined as

$$\log\left(\lambda(a,p)\right) = f(a) + \gamma(a)p$$

which is not an extension of the main-effects model, but an extension of a particular restricted main-effects model $\log\left(\lambda(a,p)\right) = f(a)+p$. This is mostly seen in survival analysis where $f(a)$ has the role of the (log) underlying hazard function—see section 8.4 on Cox-models, p. 188.

The varying coefficients model is easily fitted using gam; the s function has a by= argument, allowing a linear component in the interaction:

```
> mgpv   <- gam( cbind(D,Y/10^5) ~ s(A,k=15) +
+                                  s(P,k=15) +
+                                  s(A,k=15,by=P), family=poisreg,
                                  data=tdk )
> anova( mgp, mgpv, miap, test="Chisq" )
Analysis of Deviance Table

Model 1: cbind(D, Y/10^5) ~ s(A, k = 15) + s(P, k = 5)
Model 2: cbind(D, Y/10^5) ~ s(A, k = 15) + s(P, k = 15) + s(A, k = 15,
    by = P)
Model 3: cbind(D, Y/10^5) ~ s(A, P, k = 50)
  Resid. Df Resid. Dev    Df Deviance  Pr(>Chi)
1    2684.3     2941.8
```

```
2    2682.9      2905.7  1.4546    36.131 5.083e-09
3    2654.3      2829.5 28.5317    76.115 3.308e-06
> c( ap=mgp$aic, apv=mgpv$aic, iap=miap$aic )
      ap       apv       iap
9422.079 9388.394 9360.989
```

CODE EXPLAINED: When we use the argument by=P for a quantitative (i.e. numerical, non-factor) variable in s in a gam, we estimate in a model where the coefficient to P varies by A, as described above. To be sure to capture the non-linearity we set the initial number of knots (k) to 15 for all three effects.

In addition to the anova that compares the models by likelihood-ratio tests, we also compare the models using the AIC.

From the anova, we see that the difference in deviance between the varying coefficient model and the main-effects model is much smaller than the difference to the full interaction model. But also that it only requires 1.4 degrees of freedom, as opposed to the 28.5 for the full interaction.

The code needed to show the age-specific incidence curves at different calendar times is the same as above—no matter the model we are still just making predictions for A-slices at different dates:

```
> yr <- seq(1950, 1990, 8)
> cl <- gray( seq(0.8, 0.1, length=6) )
> nd <- data.frame( A=seq(15, 65, 0.5) )
> plot( NA, log="y", ylim=c(0.5, 30), xlim=c(15, 65),
+         xlab="Age at FU",
+         ylab="Incidence rate per 100,000 PY" )
> for( i in 1:6 )
+   {
+ nd$P <- yr[i]
+ matshade( nd$A, ci.pred(mgpv,nd), col=cl[i] )
+   }
> text(65, 30*0.85^(5:0), yr, adj=1, col=cl)
> wh.a <- c(30:32, 31:33)
> text( wh.a, ci.pred( mgpv, data.frame(A=wh.a,P=yr) )[,1],
+       yr, cex=0.6 )
```

Slicing the surface in the other direction, showing incidence rates at selected ages (A) as a function of calendar time (P), shows the character of the varying coefficients model. All curves in the calendar time direction have the same shape (Figure 6.14); the difference between any two of these is constrained to be a linear function of time, but the slope of this difference depends on which two ages we compare:

```
> ag <- seq(15,65,10)
> cl <- gray(seq(.7,.1,length=6))
> nd <- data.frame( P=seq(1945,1995,0.5) )
> plot( NA, log="y", ylim=c(0.5,30), xlim=c(1945,1995),
+         xlab="Date of FU", ylab="Incidence rate per 100,000 PY" )
> for( i in 1:6 )
+   {
+ nd$A <- ag[i]
+ matshade( nd$P, ci.pred(mgpv,nd), col=cl[i], lwd=2 )
```

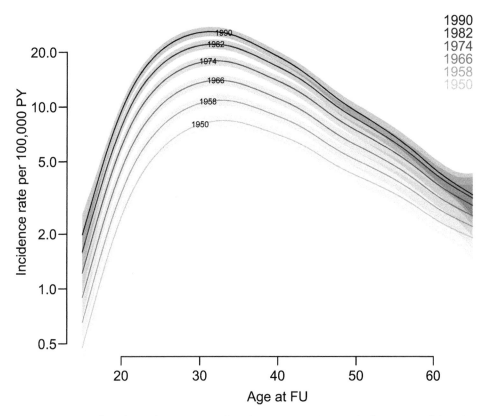

Figure 6.14 Predicted incidence rates of testis cancer in Denmark from a model with an age-varying effect of P. Each curve represents the age-specific rates at a given date; 1950-1-1, 1958-1-1, etc.

```
+     }
> text( 1945, 30*0.85^(5:0), ag, adj=0, col=cl )
>˙wh.p <- 1984
> text( wh.p, ci.pred(mgpv,data.frame(A=ag,P=wh.p))[,1],
+       ag, cex=0.6 )
```

We may illustrate the linear restriction by computing the rate ratio by calendar time between ages 15 through 65 relative to age 35 (Figure 6.15):

```
> pp <- 1943:1998
> ap <- seq(15,65,5)
> nr <- data.frame( P=pp, A=ap[5] )
> plot( NA, log="y", ylim=c(0.05,1), xlim=c(1945,1995),
+         xlab="Date of FU", ylab="RR relative to age 35" )
> for( aa in ap[-5] )
+     {
+     nd <- data.frame( P=pp, A=aa )
+     rr <- ci.exp( mgpv, list(nd,nr) )
+     matshade( pp, rr, col=gray(aa/75), lwd=2 )
+     text( 1960, rr[18,1], aa, cex=0.6 )
+     }
```

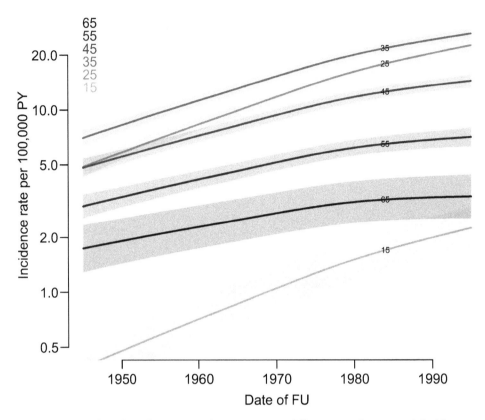

Figure 6.15 Predicted incidence rates of testis cancer in different ages from a model with an age-varying *linear* effect of date of follow-up. For each age the shape by calendar time is the same; the difference between any two curves is a linear function of the date of follow-up.

CODE EXPLAINED: We first define the *x*-axis points in `pp` and then the ages, `ap`, which we will compare to the reference age, 35 (the 5th element in `ap`). Using this as the reference we define the data frame for the predictions we will compare to, `nr`. Then we plot an empty graph, with logarithmic *y*-axis and appropriate labelling. The `for` loop runs through all the ages except the reference and computes the rate ratio.

This uses the feature of supplying a list of two data frames as the second argument to `ci.exp`; it will compute the rate ratio between the two sets of predictions based on `nd` and `nr`. These RRs are then plotted versus `pp`. The ages run from 15 to 65, so dividing by 75 (`aa/75`), we get numbers between 0 and 1 that we use to define grey tones for plotting the lines.

Finally, we annotate the lines with the age—1960 is the 18th entry of the predicted RRs in `rr`.

From Figure 6.16 we see that the slopes of the lines for ages under 35 are positive, and slopes for persons over 35 are negative. This means that the *relative* slopes seem to be declining by age, consistent with the impression from Figure 6.14, where we see the steepest increase in rates among the youngest.

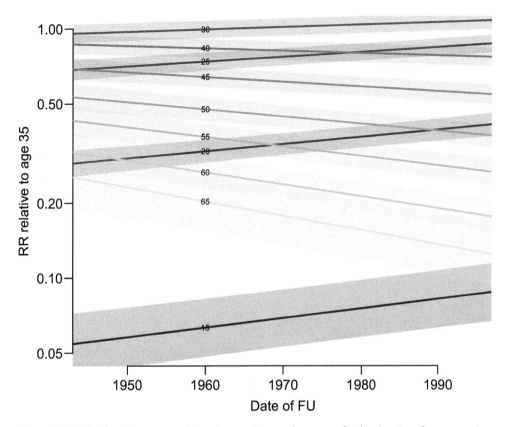

Figure 6.16 RR of testis cancer relative to age 35 as a function of calendar time from a varying coefficients model.

This phenomenon is *not* a feature of the model; the assumption in the varying coefficients model is that the curves in Figure 6.16 all are straight lines (log-RRs are linear functions of calendar time), but in the model there is no assumption about the variation in the intercept and slopes of the lines, except that they are smooth functions of age.

So it is a feature of testis cancer occurrence in Denmark that it increases more for the young and less for the old. But note that Figure 6.16 is merely an illustration of a feature of the particular chosen form of the interaction, and not particularly suited to conveying the nature of the interaction. Again, this is best done by the sliced Figures 6.14 and 6.15.

6.6.5 *Summary of quantitative interactions*

When dealing with simultaneous effects of two quantitative variables *A* and *B*, say:

1. Make sure there is some degree of independent variation in *A* and *B*—if they are closely correlated estimation of interactions is not feasible.
2. Only look for interactions you can explain.
3. Clarify if you want to show the effect of *A* for select values of *B* or vice versa, or both.
4. Do not plot predictions outside the range of data.

5. Three-dimensional surface plots are rarely useful in understanding interactions.

6. Heatmap plots can be useful in understanding interactions but they do not support confidence intervals.

7. Varying coefficients models may be a viable simplification of interactions in some circumstances, but you need to check the models against general interaction models.

In summary, interactions should be reported by predicted values in slices along both variables.

CHAPTER 7

Case-control and case-cohort studies

In a case-control study we sample persons based on their disease outcome, so the fraction of diseased persons in a case-control study is usually known (at least approximately) before data collection.

The rationale of a case-control study is as follows: sample 200 persons with malignant melanoma (cases) and 200 persons without (controls). Then determine their hair colour. If it turns out that 10% of the melanoma cases have red hair, but only 5% of the controls we would say that persons with red hair are twice as likely to contract malignant melanoma as persons with other hair colours.

This is not quite right, but pretty close—here are some bogus numbers illustrating this point:

```
> library(Epi)
> mm <- cbind( c(20,180), c(10,190) )
> colnames(mm) <- c("ca","co")
> rownames(mm) <- c("red","oth")
> mm
     ca  co
red  20  10
oth 180 190
> twoby2(mm)
2 by 2 table analysis:
------------------------------------------------
Outcome   : ca
Comparing : red vs. oth

     ca  co   P(ca) 95% conf. interval
red  20  10  0.6667    0.4835    0.8103
oth 180 190  0.4865    0.4359    0.5374

                                95% conf. interval
            Relative Risk: 1.3704    1.0421    1.8020
        Sample Odds Ratio: 2.1111    0.9620    4.6330
Conditional MLE Odds Ratio: 2.1073    0.9120    5.1859
   Probability difference: 0.1802   -0.0058    0.3300


            Exact P-value: 0.0861
       Asymptotic P-value: 0.0624
------------------------------------------------
```

Epidemiology with R. Bendix Carstensen, Oxford University Press (2021). © Bendix Carstensen.
DOI: 10.1093/oso/9780198841326.003.0008

> CODE EXPLAINED: The 2 by 2 table of exposure by case-control status should have cases in the first column and exposed in the first row when used as input to `twoby2`. The function computes a number of common measures of association, but in a case-control setting it is only the odds ratios that are of interest. As suggested in the hand-waving, we find that the odds ratio of malignant melanoma when comparing red-haired to other is about 2.

But first let us get the quantitative concepts hammered out in more detail.

7.1 Follow-up and case-control studies

In a cohort (follow-up) study, the relationship between some exposure and disease incidence is investigated by following the entire cohort and measuring the rate of occurrence of new cases in the different exposure groups. The follow-up records all persons who develop the disease during the study period. Implicit in this is that the relevant exposure information is available at all times for *all* persons under follow-up. For simplicity we shall start by assuming that there are two types of persons—exposed and non-exposed, that is, a binary exposure variable.

In a case-control study the persons who develop the disease (the cases) are registered by some other mechanism than follow-up—typically, a disease register, or hospital records. A group of healthy persons (the controls) is used to represent the persons who do not develop the disease. When cases and controls have been identified, *then* the relevant exposure information is collected. Thus information collection is retrospective; this is why a case-control study occasionally (particularly in older literature) is referred to as a 'retrospective study'.

In a simple follow-up study where only exposure or not is considered, rates among exposed (1) and non-exposed (0) are estimated by

$$\frac{D_1}{Y_1} \quad \text{resp.} \quad \frac{D_0}{Y_0}$$

Where D are cases and Y are Person-years; and hence the rate ratio by

$$\text{RR} = \frac{D_1}{Y_1} \bigg/ \frac{D_0}{Y_0} = \frac{D_1}{D_0} \bigg/ \frac{Y_1}{Y_0}$$

As noted earlier, in cohort studies we assume that all covariate information is available for all persons in the cohort—in this simplified example the only covariate is whether a person is exposed. Usually, collecting covariate information is expensive in a cohort study, because it must be collected for all persons in the cohort.

The rearrangement of the expression for the rate ratio shows that the quantities we need are the ratio between the exposed and unexposed cases and the ratio between the exposed and unexposed person-years. But it is only the latter which is expensive to collect because it involves information from the entire cohort. In the case-control study we use a sample from the non-diseased to get an estimate of the ratio of exposed to non-exposed person-years through the ratio of exposed to non-exposed controls, so if we choose controls as representative of the person-years in the cohort, we obtain after classifying them (H_1 as exposed and H_0 as unexposed)

$$\frac{H_1}{H_0} \approx \frac{Y_1}{Y_0}$$

and so therefore the rate ratio in the population can be estimated by

$$\frac{D_1}{D_0} \Big/ \frac{H_1}{H_0}$$

The economic point here is that we need not collect covariate (i.e. exposure) information from the entire population, but only from the cases and a limited number of controls.

If *all* variables needed in the analysis are available at no extra cost for the entire population (cohort) there is no need to do a case-control study; the only effect of doing a case-control study would be to lose the possibility of estimating the *absolute* occurrence rates (and a slight loss of precision in estimating RRs).

7.1.1 *Probabilities and odds in case-control studies*

We can illustrate the selection machinery for cases and controls while keeping track of the probabilities we are after; see Figure 7.1. Suppose we have a fixed study period, in which the fraction of exposed individuals is p throughout the period, and in which the probability of acquiring the disease in the study period among exposed and non-exposed is π_1, resp. π_0. Further, let the sampling fractions (the probability that a person is included in the study) be s_0 and s_1 for un-exposed and exposed cases, respectively, and similarly k_0 and k_1 for controls. Typically, the sampling fractions for cases s_0 and s_1 will be close to 1 because we take almost all cases into the study, whereas the sampling fractions k_0 and k_1 for the controls will be very small.

The sampling fractions for exposed and un-exposed must be equal, but we keep them as separate entities here in order to illustrate precisely where the assumption of equality is crucial.

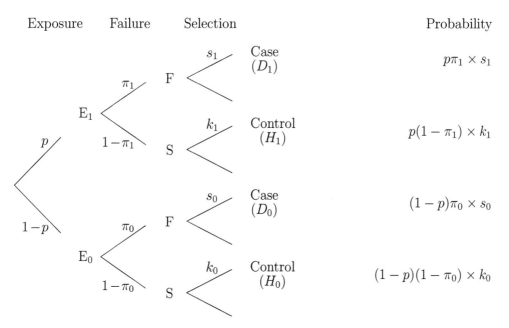

Figure 7.1 Probability tree illustrating selection of cases and controls. p is the exposure probability in the population, π_0 the disease probability in unexposed, and π_1 the disease probability in exposed. The s and k are sampling probabilities (see text).

These quantities are illustrated in the probability tree in Figure 7.1; it shows what goes on in the *entire* population. The first split of the population is according to exposure; p of the population is exposed, $1 - p$ is not. The next is disease occurrence, with disease probabilities π_1 for exposed and π_0 for non-exposed. The final split is by inclusion in the study, where we only see those included in the study according to the inclusion probabilities (sampling fractions). On the right are the probabilities that a random person from the population will enter the study as e.g. exposed control. These are products of the (conditional) probabilities shown on the branches of the probability tree.

Note that the four probabilities on the right in Figure 7.1 do not sum to 1; the sum of them is the probability that a person from the population is included in the study.

If we look at the disease *odds*, ω (given inclusion in the study), we have for exposed and un-exposed:

$$\left(\frac{D_1}{H_1} \approx\right) \; \omega_1 \;=\; \frac{p s_1 \pi_1}{p k_1 (1 - \pi_1)} \;=\; \frac{s_1 \pi_1}{k_1 (1 - \pi_1)} \;=\; \frac{s_1}{k_1} \times \frac{\pi_1}{1 - \pi_1}$$

$$\left(\frac{D_0}{H_0} \approx\right) \; \omega_0 \;=\; \frac{(1 - p) s_0 \pi_0}{(1 - p) k_0 (1 - \pi_0)} \;=\; \frac{s_0 \pi_0}{k_0 (1 - \pi_0)} \;=\; \frac{s_0}{k_0} \times \frac{\pi_0}{1 - \pi_0}$$

which means that the disease *ratio* between exposed and non-exposed, *given inclusion in the study*, is

$$\mathrm{OR}_{\text{study}} = \frac{D_1/H_1}{D_0/H_0} \approx \frac{s_1/k_1 \times \pi_1/(1 - \pi_1)}{s_0/k_0 \times \pi_0/(1 - \pi_0)} = \frac{\pi_1/(1 - \pi_1)}{\pi_0/(1 - \pi_0)} = \mathrm{OR}_{\text{population}}$$

Note that the penultimate '=' in the formula is only correct if the sampling fractions do not depend on exposure status, that is, if $s_0 = s_1$ and $k_0 = k_1$. So the inclusion of persons in a case-control study must be independent of exposure status—in general independent of any covariate whose effect we want to quantify. If this is not the case the assertion that the *study* OR is the same as the *population* OR breaks down.

7.1.2 The sampling fractions

Note that we do not need to know the sampling fractions, we just need to know that they do not depend on exposure status (i.e. on any of the covariates of interest). Normally the design of a case-control study will be to include as many cases as possible, so that s will be close to 1. The number of controls included will often be determined in some way by the (anticipated) number of cases. So in neither case do we know what the sampling fractions are, but we will not need them either.

7.1.3 A simple example

We can illustrate this using the `lep` dataset of a case-control study of leprosy in Tanzania (use `?lep` for more details):

```
> library( Epi )
> data( lep )
> ( cctab <- with( lep, table( bcg, factor(d,labels=c("Co","Ca")) ) ) )
bcg    Co   Ca
  no   596 227
  yes  500  47
> ( do <- cctab[,"Ca"]/cctab[,"Co"] )
```

```
         no         yes
0.3808725 0.0940000
> ( OR <- do["yes"]/do["no"] )
      yes
0.2468018
```

> CODE EXPLAINED: The variable d is numeric coded 0 for controls and 1 for cases, so when we use it as a factor the `labels` argument to `factor` must list controls before cases because $0 < 1$. `bcg` is already a factor. Note that we have placed brackets around the assignments to have the results listed.
>
> `do` is the disease odds—the `Ca` column of `cctab` divided by the `Co` column. The odds ratio (`OR`) is computed as the ratio of the two resulting disease odds; note that we can refer to the elements of the vectors and tables by name, so the calculations are independent of how the levels of disease and exposure are ordered, but most importantly, the resulting code becomes closer to being human readable.

We see that children with a BCG scar (meaning they have been vaccinated against tuberculosis) have about a quarter of the risk of leprosy as those without.

7.2 Statistical model for the odds ratio

If we want confidence intervals for odds and odds ratios we must resort to a proper statistical model. The observations we have are the number of cases and controls, that is, a binary outcome (case/control), one set for each exposure group, D cases and H controls.

Recall from Chapter 3 (formula 3.1, p. 50) that the standard error of the log-odds for x events out of a total of n possible was $\sqrt{1/x + 1/(n-x)}$. We have D successes out of $D + H$, so the standard error of the log disease odds, $\log(\omega) = \log(D/H)$ is

$$\text{s.e.}\left(\log(\omega)\right) = \sqrt{\frac{1}{D} + \frac{1}{H}} \quad \Leftrightarrow \quad \text{var}\left(\log(\omega)\right) = \frac{1}{D} + \frac{1}{H}$$

The same goes for both exposed and un-exposed, and since they are independent bodies of data, the variance of the log-odds ratio (which is the difference of the log-odds) is the sum of the variances of the log-odds, so

$$\text{s.e.}\left(\log(\text{OR})\right) = \sqrt{\frac{1}{D_0} + \frac{1}{H_0} + \frac{1}{D_1} + \frac{1}{H_1}}$$

The way to compute a confidence interval for the OR is first to do it on the log-scale:

$$\log(\text{OR}) \pm 1.96\sqrt{\frac{1}{D_0} + \frac{1}{H_0} + \frac{1}{D_1} + \frac{1}{H_1}}$$

and then back-transform

$$\text{OR} \overset{\times}{\div} \exp\left(1.96\sqrt{\frac{1}{D_0} + \frac{1}{H_0} + \frac{1}{D_1} + \frac{1}{H_1}}\right)$$

This formula (and quite a few others) are implemented in the `twoby2` function used in the beginning of this chapter.

We may also use the function `effx` which will do the calculation directly on the original dataset with the individual records, and provide an easily read summary. Beside the dataset (`data=lep`), we must specify the name and type of the response variable, and the name of the exposure variable:

```
> effx( response = d,
+           type = 'binary',
+       exposure = bcg,
+           data = lep )

---------------------------------------------------------------

response     :   d
type         :   binary
exposure     :   bcg

bcg is a factor with levels: no / yes
baseline is   no
effects are measured as odds ratios
---------------------------------------------------------------


effect of bcg on d
number of observations   1370

Effect    2.5%   97.5%
 0.247   0.176   0.345

Test for no effects of exposure on 1 df: p-value= <2e-16
```

7.2.1 *Analysis by logistic regression*

When we set up a statistical model we must do this for the disease process that we are interested in, at the *population* level. For the sake of generality we assume we have a variable x_1 and we want to use our case-control study to assess the effect of it on disease occurrence. Since the case-control setup only allows for estimating effects on the odds-ratio-scale, we assume that the relationship between the disease probability π (referring to some study period) and exposure x_1 in the population is

$$\log\left[\frac{\pi}{1-\pi}\right] = \beta_0 + \beta_1 x_1$$

In our leprosy example we had $x_1 = 1$ for persons with a BCG scar and $x_1 = 0$ for persons without. Hence the log disease odds for persons without BCG scar is β_0 and for persons with a BCG scar $\beta_0 + \beta_1 x_1$, and so the log disease odds ratio between a person with and one without a BCG scar is $\beta_1 x_1$.

In general, it means that the log of the disease odds ratio between two persons that differ 1 in the variable x_1 is $\beta_0 + \beta_1(x+1) - (\beta_0 + \beta_1 x) = \beta_1$, so e^{β_1} is the odds ratio associated with a difference of 1 in the covariate x_1.

But we do not observe disease occurrence in the *population*; we sampled, so we must use the *conditional* probability, *given* that a person is included in the study, because this is what we observed. Assuming the sampling fractions to be s and k for cases and controls respectively, we saw earlier that the disease odds in the model was the population odds multiplied by the ratio of the sampling fractions:

$$\log(\text{odds}(\text{case}|\text{incl.})) = \log\left[\frac{\pi}{1-\pi} \times \frac{s}{k}\right] = \log\left[\frac{\pi}{1-\pi}\right] + \log\left[\frac{s}{k}\right]$$

$$= \left(\log\left[\frac{s}{k}\right] + \beta_0\right) + \beta_1 x_1 \tag{7.1}$$

So we see that the effect of our exposure variable will be estimated correctly if we model the *study* disease odds *as if* they were population odds. The price we pay for not having true population data is that the intercept in the model is meaningless because it involves the ratio of the sampling fractions, which are usually not known—remember?

This means that in `glm` we just use the data as if they were population observations:

```
> x <- 0:1
> ca <- cctab[,"Ca"]
> co <- cctab[,"Co"]
> cbind( ca, co, x )
     ca  co x
no  227 596 0
yes  47 500 1
> mg <- glm( cbind(ca,co) ~ x, family=binomial )
> round( ci.exp( mg ), 3 )
            exp(Est.)  2.5% 97.5%
(Intercept)     0.381 0.327 0.444
x               0.247 0.176 0.345
```

> CODE EXPLAINED: For logistic regression with R we need two vectors, one with the cases (`ca`) and one with the controls (`co`), so they are extracted from `cctab`. The `glm` with `family=binomial` fits the logistic regression model. Since the intercept is meaningless, it will not be sensible to make predictions from either the model or the models for the prevalences in Chapter 3. The response variable (the l.h.s. of '~') is just a 2-column matrix with the first column cases and the second controls, so instead we could have used directly `glm(cctab[,2:1]~x,family=binomial)`, or for the sake of readability `glm(cctab[,c("Ca","Co")]~x,family=binomial)`
>
> The function `ci.exp` extracts the parameters and confidence intervals and exponentiates them—also the meaningless intercept—there is no way the program can tell that this is a case-control study and not a prevalence study, where the intercept indeed would have been meaningful.

We see that we get the same estimate we got from `effx` (OR = 0.247). As in the analysis by `effx`, we may use `glm` directly on the individual records. In fact `effx` uses `glm` internally. In this case we can just use the *numerical* 0/1 variable `d` as the response variable:

```
> mi <- glm( d ~ bcg, family=binomial, data=lep )
> round( ci.exp( mi ), 3 )
            exp(Est.)  2.5% 97.5%
(Intercept)     0.381 0.327 0.444
bcgyes          0.247 0.176 0.345
```

> CODE EXPLAINED: We use the binary variable `d` as the response variable, modelling the probability of seeing the value 1.[1] Note that we can use `d` and `bcg` directly; the `data=lep` argument tells R to look for the variables in the `lep` data frame.

The estimate indicates that persons with a BCG scar have a risk of leprosy which is about a quarter of that for persons without a BCG scar.

---

[1] `glm` actually also allows a `factor` to be the response variable, in which case the *first* level is taken as 0 and the union of the remaining levels as 1. In code, if the response is the factor `ff`, the result will be as if we used `(ff != levels(ff)[1])*1` as a numerical response. Not recommended—it makes your code difficult to read.

7.3 Odds ratio and rate ratio

What we are estimating from a case-control study is the ratio of disease odds referring to some study period of length ℓ, say. If the study period is short in the sense that the disease probability over the period is small, then we have the approximation for the odds ratio,

$$\text{OR} = \frac{\pi_1}{1-\pi_1} \bigg/ \frac{\pi_0}{1-\pi_0} \approx \pi_1/\pi_0 = \lambda_1\ell/\lambda_0\ell = \lambda_1/\lambda_0 = \text{RR}$$

where λ_1 and λ_0 are the occurrence rates—assumed constant over the study period. Note that the essential assumption in the approximation is that $(1 - \pi_1)/(1 - \pi_0) \approx 1$; this is a very accurate approximation if both π_1 and π_0 are close to 0.

With the assumption of a small probability we therefore have that the odds ratio is a reasonable *estimate* of the rate ratio.

7.3.1 *Incidence density sampling*

If we sample controls by selecting one or more from the population every time a case occurs, we may think of the total case-control study as many *very* short case-control studies, each with one case (or very few). For each of these, the above approximation of the OR to the RR will be accurate because the study duration is small, and hence the core part of the approximation becomes more accurate.

These short studies can then be analysed as one under the assumption that there is no trend in the prevalence of exposure over the study period.

So if the sampling of controls is carried out as incidence density sampling the odds ratio computed from the case-control study is a good estimate of the population rate ratio.

7.4 Confounding and stratified sampling

If we anticipate confounding by some variable, we want to include this in the model. Recall (see p. 30) that if a variable is associated with both the exposure of interest and the disease outcome (and is assumed not to be on the causal path from exposure to outcome) we may get a distorted estimate of the exposure effect. The solution is to include the confounding variable as the explanatory variable in the model. That will produce an estimate of the exposure effect *conditional* on the value of the confounding variable—under the assumption that the exposure effect is the same across the range of the confounding variable. This is a basic assumption when including a variable in a regression model.

Because the confounding variable is associated both with the outcome and the exposure, a dataset with randomly sampled controls may turn out with a lot of controls and very few cases for some values of the confounder, and vice versa for other values of the confounder. Since the major argument for conducting a case-control study is saving money in the data-collection process, this wasteful data collection would be quite silly. There are two ways used to remedy this: (1) stratified sampling and (2) matched sampling.

7.4.1 *Stratified sampling*

In this case, controls are sampled within *strata* of the potential confounder, such that the ratio of the number of controls relative to the number of cases is the same in each stratum. This has the effect that the sampling fractions s and k are not the same in different strata. So we are conducting a separate case-control study in each stratum, with different sampling fractions in each stratum.

Therefore, looking at Eq. (7.1) for logistic regression of the ratio of the sampling fractions (s/k) varies between strata, and hence this must be accommodated in the model—we have a different intercept for each stratum. This means that we must include the stratifying variable as a *factor* in the model if data are sampled separately in each stratum.

As an illustration of this machinery we make a 1:1 stratified sample from the `lep` data across the ageclasses, and compare it with a similar random sample of the same number of persons. We use the very simple `matchControls` function from the `e1071` package:

```
> set.seed( 1952 ) # to ensure reproducibility
> library(e1071)
> str( whcc <- matchControls( d ~ age,  data=lep, case=1, cont=0 ) )
List of 3
 $ cases   : chr [1:274] "5" "9" "10" "11" ...
 $ controls: chr [1:274] "1221" "840" "736" "1145" ...
 $ factor  : Factor w/ 2 levels "case","cont": NA NA NA NA 1 NA NA 2 1 1 ...
  ..- attr(*, "names")= chr [1:1370] "1" "2" "3" "4" ...
> mlep <- subset( lep, !is.na(whcc$factor) )
```

CODE EXPLAINED: The `matchControls` returns a list, where the 3rd element is a factor, called `factor`, of the same length as the number of rows in `lep`. This has levels case or control for the matched cases and controls, and is missing for those not matched to cases (cases are those coded as 1 in the l.h.s. variable in the formula, here the variable d). So if we discard those with missing values (`!is.na(whcc$factor)`), we have a stratified study with an equal number of cases and controls. This is in the data frame `mlep`.

```
> ca <- subset( lep, d==1 )
> co <- subset( lep, d==0 )
> co <- co[sample(nrow(co),nrow(ca)),]
> rlep <- rbind( ca, co )
```

CODE EXPLAINED: `ca` is the subset of `lep` consisting of all cases and `co` the subset consisting of all controls.

The data frame `rlep` is made by taking all cases (`ca`) and a random sample of the controls—the function `sample(N,n)` returns a random sample of size n of the numbers `1:N`. So what is done is simply to select a random set of the controls of the same size as the set of cases. This is then put head-to-foot with the cases (`rbind`) to form the dataset `rlep`.

```
> cbind( with( mlep, addmargins( table(age, d) ) ),
+       with( rlep, addmargins( table(age, d) ) ) )
```

	0	1	Sum	0	1	Sum
5-9	34	34	68	70	34	104
10-14	35	35	70	56	35	91
15-19	21	21	42	37	21	58
20-24	18	18	36	22	18	40
25-29	31	31	62	15	31	46
30-44	64	64	128	39	64	103

```
45+     71   71 142   35   71 106
Sum    274 274 548  274  274 548
```

> CODE EXPLAINED: We then tabulate case-control status versus age in the two constructed case-control studies, use `addmargins` to put margins on the tables, and finally print them side by side.

Once we have these two artificial case-control datasets we can estimate the effect of `bcg` from both of them, both ignoring and including the confounder `age`.

```
> mm.0 <- glm( d ~ bcg        , family=binomial, data=mlep )
> mm.a <- glm( d ~ bcg + age, family=binomial, data=mlep )
> rm.0 <- glm( d ~ bcg        , family=binomial, data=rlep )
> rm.a <- glm( d ~ bcg + age, family=binomial, data=rlep )
> or <- rbind( ci.exp(mm.0,subset="bcg"),
+               ci.exp(mm.a,subset="bcg"),
+               ci.exp(rm.0,subset="bcg"),
+               ci.exp(rm.a,subset="bcg") )
> rownames( or ) <- c("mm.0","mm.a","rm.0","rm.a")
> or
      exp(Est.)      2.5%      97.5%
mm.0 0.4450352 0.2970747 0.6666886
mm.a 0.3363147 0.2091196 0.5408748
rm.0 0.2657122 0.1790986 0.3942129
rm.a 0.3738019 0.2390489 0.5845157
> plotEst( or, lwd=2, xlog=TRUE, grid=1:10/10, vref=1 )
```

> CODE EXPLAINED: The first 4 lines fit logistic regression models; it is only those with age included that give unbiased (un-confounded) estimates. We use `ci.exp` to extract the OR associated with `bcg`, and stack these in a matrix using `rbind`. The `anova` command uses likelihood-ratio tests to compare models. Finally, the `plotEst` plots estimate with confidence limits from the matrix of ORs; `lwd` determines the width of the lines indicating the confidence intervals; `xlog=TRUE` gives a logarithmic x-axis; `grid=` defines vertical grid lines; and `vref=1` puts a vertical reference line at 1. See `?plotEst` for further arguments.

We see that the two sets of estimates from models controlling for age are pretty close but also that they have wider confidence intervals than the ones ignoring age. The estimates ignoring the confounder (age) obtain the narrower confidence intervals from making the (wrong) assumption of no confounding by age.

We can make formal tests of the effect of `age` by comparing the models with and without age included:

```
> anova( mm.a, mm.0, test="Chisq" )
Analysis of Deviance Table

Model 1: d ~ bcg + age
Model 2: d ~ bcg
  Resid. Df Resid. Dev Df Deviance Pr(>Chi)
1       540     738.31
2       546     743.69 -6  -5.3886    0.495
```

```
> anova( rm.a, rm.0, test="Chisq" )
Analysis of Deviance Table

Model 1: d ~ bcg + age
Model 2: d ~ bcg
  Resid. Df Resid. Dev Df Deviance Pr(>Chi)
1       540     693.73
2       546     712.60 -6  -18.876 0.004378
```

> CODE EXPLAINED: The anova function with the argument test="Chisq" compares models
> via the log-likelihood ratio. Models must be fitted to the same data, and must be nested
> (that is, one model must be a sub-model of the other; see section 3.3.1, p. 60), so it is
> meaningless to compare any of the mm models to any of the mr models, because they are
> fitted to different datasets.

From the tests of the models using anova, we see that the test for age in the matched
models is non-significant; however; this is a meaningless test. The variable we are
addressing, age, was used as stratification in a stratified sampled study, so the outcome
will necessarily be balanced across ages and thus the test will produce a very high p-value.
On the other hand, omitting it from the model induces bias, because we must account
for the different sampling fractions in different strata. The test for age-effect in the study
based on a *random* sample of controls *is*, however, meaningful, and including age in the
model not only shows a strong age-effect, but also substantial influence on the estimate
of the BCG effect when included in the model.

Omitting the stratification variable from the model will usually lead to a dilution of
the exposure effect—this is seen from the two upper estimates in Figure 7.2, where the
estimate from the model mm.0 without the stratification variable is closer to 1 relative
to the estimate from model mm.a. The confounding by age in the analysis based on a
randomly sampled study can go in any direction; in this case, the confounded estimate
(from model rm.0) is further away from 1 then the correct one (from model rm.a)

Thus the conclusion is that you must always include the confounder in the model, also
when you have a stratified sampling design. Testing for the effect of a variable used for

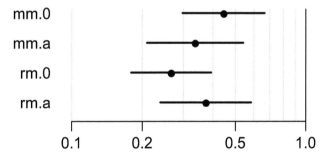

Figure 7.2 Odds ratios of leprosy associated with the presence
of a BCG scar from stratified and random sampling of controls.
The two top estimates are based on the stratified data, the
two bottom ones on a random sample of controls of the same
size as cases. Models with a '.0' are models ignoring the age
variable (age), while models with a '.a' are models where age
is included in the model.

stratification of your case-control data is meaningless, but the variable should be included in the model nevertheless.

7.5 Individually matched studies

In the example we just saw the sample was stratified on age, using seven 5-year age groups, so in each stratum there were several cases and controls, and the number of strata was limited. And the inclusion of the age group in the model required 6 extra parameters.

If we (in the sampling design) want to control for a confounder that takes a lot of values and which might not even be quantifiable—such as place of residence and/or education—the number of strata might be very large and each stratum might contain only 1 case and a small number of controls.

It turns out that in such a design, the conventional statistics breaks down because the number of stratum parameters is proportional to the study size (number of cases), loosely speaking 'almost as big as' the number of cases. This means that we will get biased effect estimates if we use ordinary logistic regression. The solution is to use the *conditional* likelihood *given* the number of cases and controls in each stratum.

The underlying assumption behind this reasoning is that in each matched set (stratum) s, say, the disease odds for individual i in the stratum is a product of a stratum effect ω_s and an individual effect θ_i:

$$\text{odds(disease)} = \omega_s \theta_i \quad \Leftrightarrow \quad \text{P\{disease\}} = \frac{\omega_s \theta_i}{1 + \omega_s \theta_i} \quad \Leftrightarrow \quad \text{P\{no disease\}} = \frac{1}{1 + \omega_s \theta_i}$$

The θ_i is the term that depends on the individual-level covariates such as exposure, whereas the ω_s is the contribution to disease probability from factors common for all persons in matched set s. We are not really interested in the latter, and hence refer to them as *nuisance* parameters.

Suppose we have 3 persons (one case and two controls), a, b, and c in a matched set—based on the set (s) and covariates; the disease odds for the three persons are then

$$a : \omega_a = \omega_s \theta_a, \qquad b : \omega_b = \omega_s \theta_b, \qquad c : \omega_c = \omega_s \theta_c$$

The sampling design is such that one of these is a case and the other two are controls. The likelihood is the probability of data, *conditional* on design, i.e. on 1 case and 2 controls in the matched set. The information about the relationship between exposure (covariates) and disease is in the differences in distribution of covariates for the case and the controls.

If person a is the case and b and c the controls, the likelihood contribution from matched set s is

$$L = \text{P\{}a \text{ is case} \mid 1 \text{ case, 2 con among } a, b, c\}$$

$$= \frac{\text{P\{}a \text{ is case} \mid b, c \text{ con}\}}{\text{P\{}a \text{ is case} \mid b, c \text{ con}\} + \text{P\{}b \text{ is case} \mid a, c \text{ con}\} + \text{P\{}c \text{ is case} \mid a, b \text{ con}\}}$$

$$= \frac{\omega_a/(1 + \omega_a) \times 1/(1 + \omega_b) \times 1/(1 + \omega_c))}{(\omega_a + \omega_b + \omega_c)/((1 + \omega_a)(1 + \omega_b)(1 + \omega_c))}$$

$$= \frac{\omega_a}{\omega_a + \omega_b + \omega_c} = \frac{\omega_s \theta_a}{\omega_s \theta_a + \omega_s \theta_b + \omega_s \theta_c} = \frac{\theta_a}{\theta_a + \theta_b + \theta_c}$$

The thing to note here is that because we condition on the sampling scheme each stratum (1 case, 2 controls), the contribution to the likelihood does not depend on the set-specific parameter ω_s. This means that when we fit models, there will be no intercept parameter as in traditional regression models.

In general, with one case and a number of controls, the conditional likelihood contribution from one matched set is the *conditional* probability that person a is the case and persons $b, c, \dots$ are the controls, *given* that there is one case and (say) m controls in the matched set:

$$\ell = \frac{\theta_{case}}{\sum_{i \in \text{cases \& controls}} \theta_i}$$

This formula easily generalizes to more than 2 controls per case, and no assumption about the same number of controls in each matched set is needed. The log-likelihood for the total study is

$$\ell = \sum_{\text{matched sets}} \log \left(\frac{\theta_{case}}{\sum_{i \in \text{cases \& controls}} \theta_i} \right)$$

This very closely resembles the log-likelihood for a stratified Cox-model from a dataset where each case dies before the controls (see section 8.4), so it will be no surprise that the function `clogit` that will analyse data using *conditional logistic regression* is from the `survival` package.

A slightly (well, much) more complicated formula is available for the situation where there are more than one *case* in each matched set, say 2 cases and 3 controls. This is also implemented in the functions `clogit` from the `survival` package and `clogistic` from the `Epi` package, the latter in a somewhat more efficient version for the situation with more than 1 case per matched set.

7.5.1 *An example*

As an example we use the 1:4 matched case-control study where women with endometrial cancer each were matched to 4 women without the disease on age, marital status, and place of residence. The exposure of interest is former conjugated estrogen therapy in the variable `est` (yes/no) and the duration of this in the variable `dur` (0,1,2,3,4). The matched set variable is `set`:

```
> library( Epi )
> library( survival )
> data( bdendo )
> head( bdendo )
  set d gall hyp    ob est dur non duration age cest agegrp   age3
1   1 1   No  No  Yes Yes   4 Yes       96  74    3 70-74 65-74
2   1 0   No  No <NA>  No   0  No        0  75    0 70-74 65-74
3   1 0   No  No <NA>  No   0  No        0  74    0 70-74 65-74
4   1 0   No  No <NA>  No   0  No        0  74    0 70-74 65-74
5   1 0   No  No  Yes Yes   3 Yes       48  75    1 70-74 65-74
6   2 1   No  No   No Yes   4 Yes       96  67    3 65-69 65-74
> ms <- clogit(     d ~ gall+hyp+est+dur+ strata(set), data=bdendo )
> mE <- clogistic( d ~ gall+hyp+est+dur, strata=set , data=bdendo )
> round( cbind( ci.exp(ms), ci.exp(mE) ), 4 )
        exp(Est.)    2.5%  97.5% exp(Est.)    2.5%   97.5%
gallYes    3.1588  1.2946 7.7075    3.1588  1.2946  7.7075
hypYes     0.7836  0.3690 1.6641    0.7836  0.3690  1.6641
```

```
estYes      6.7157 1.6722 26.9706     6.7156 1.6722 26.9705
dur1        0.7784 0.1887  3.2116     0.7784 0.1887  3.2116
dur2        1.1780 0.3360  4.1298     1.1780 0.3360  4.1298
dur3        2.5632 0.6508 10.0952     2.5632 0.6508 10.0951
dur4        2.7320 0.7589  9.8348     2.7320 0.7589  9.8348
```

> CODE EXPLAINED: The two different versions of conditional logistic regression give the same results; the major difference is in the analysis of studies with more than one case per stratum where `clogit` is ineffective (see the help page for `clogit`). For studies with only 1 case per stratum, the difference between the two is negligible.
>
> Note that there is a difference in how the stratum variable (`set` in this case) is entered in the two functions.
>
> The estimates are extracted and exponentiated by `ci.exp`, and the result are odds ratios associated with each of the variables in the model.

We see that the odds ratio of endometrial cancer associated with previous gall bladder disease is 3.2 but with a very wide confidence interval (1.3–7.7), so we cannot really tell whether the effect is rather small or very large. There is apparently no effect of hypertension, but neither a halving of the risk or a 50% increase can be excluded.

Note that the two variables `est` and `dur` are associated in the dataset:

```
> with( bdendo, table(est, dur) )
     dur
est      0   1   2   3   4
  No   132   0   0   0   0
  Yes   23  32  44  27  40
```

The reference category for the duration of estrogen, `dur`, is 0, and for the ever use of estrogen, `est`, it is No. So the rate ratio of 6.1 associated with `est` compares (Yes,0), with (No,0), whereas the rate ratio of 0.78 associated with `dur1` compares persons with duration 1 to persons with duration 0 (both with `est-Yes`).

So if we want the combined effect of the two so that we can see the rate ratio for each of the `dur` categories relative to the `est-N0` category, we must combine the estimates for `est` and `dur`. A simpler way is to use the function `interaction` that generates the interaction factor whose levels are all combinations of the two factors:

```
> with( bdendo, table( interaction(est,dur) ) )

 No.0 Yes.0  No.1 Yes.1  No.2 Yes.2  No.3 Yes.3  No.4 Yes.4
  132    23     0    32     0    44     0    27     0    40
> is <- clogit( d ~ gall + hyp +
+                        factor( interaction(est,dur) ) +
+                        strata(set),
+               data = bdendo )
> iE <- clogistic( d ~ gall + hyp + interaction(est,dur),
+                        strata = set,
+                        data = bdendo )
> ( ci.exp(is) / ci.exp(iE) )
                                    exp(Est.)        2.5%      97.5%
gallYes                             1.000001 1.0000007 1.000001
hypYes                              1.000000 0.9999999 1.000000
factor(interaction(est, dur))Yes.0 1.000003 1.0000023 1.000004
```

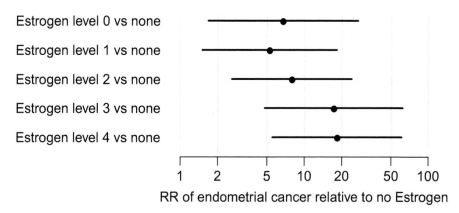

Figure 7.3 Estimates of the rate ratios for different estrogen exposure levels relative to no exposure. The dots represent the estimates, and the bars the 95% confidence intervals.

```
factor(interaction(est, dur))Yes.1  1.000003 1.0000022 1.000003
factor(interaction(est, dur))Yes.2  1.000003 1.0000022 1.000004
factor(interaction(est, dur))Yes.3  1.000003 1.0000026 1.000004
factor(interaction(est, dur))Yes.4  1.000003 1.0000025 1.000004

> ( RR <- ci.exp( iE, subset = "est" ) )

                               exp(Est.)     2.5%     97.5%
interaction(est, dur)Yes.0   6.715631 1.672184 26.97053
interaction(est, dur)Yes.1   5.227411 1.502375 18.18842
interaction(est, dur)Yes.2   7.910884 2.613438 23.94627
interaction(est, dur)Yes.3  17.213813 4.788549 61.87998
interaction(est, dur)Yes.4  18.346933 5.535879 60.80515

> rownames( RR ) <- paste( "Estrogen level", 0:4, "vs. none" )
> plotEst( RR, xlog=T, grid=TRUE,
+          xlab="RR of endometrial cancer relative to no Estrogen" )
```

CODE EXPLAINED: The interaction creates a factor with all combinations, including the empty ones. We can get rid of the empty levels by putting the result inside the factor function. This is needed inside the clogit function; otherwise, it will crash because of the empty levels. clogistic handles empty levels correctly. The estimated parameters are assigned to RR and printed by means of the brackets. For readability we use paste to generate nice labels for the parameters.

Finally, the function plotEst shows the estimates in a forest plot; the first argument to plotEst must have 3 columns, one with the estimate and two with the upper and lower limits—the argument xlog makes the x-axis logarithmic, and the grid argument draws the vertical grid lines at the tick marks. The result is in Figure 7.3.

7.5.2 *When conditional analysis is not needed*

Occasionally an individual matching is made using quantitative variables, typically using age or date of birth. In this case the model invoked above with a separate parameter ω_s for each matched set is not necessarily sensible or necessary. Since the sets are defined *only* by age, say, it would be more sensible to exploit the quantitative nature of the matching variable and use a *model* for the strata, the ω_ss. This would avoid the problems with the large number of ω_ss that in the first place lead to the necessity of the conditional approach.

In this situation we can just resort to the ordinary logistic regression approach by including a (non-linear, smooth) effect of the quantitative matching variable. The necessary assumption is that the *joint* effect of the ratio of sampling fractions (see section 7.1.2 on p. 162) as well as the effect of the matching variable varies smoothly with the matching variable.

Note that the estimated effect of the matching variable is not the population effect of the matching variable, but rather the *combined* effect of the matching variable and the variation of the sampling fractions with the matching variable—the latter normally unknown. So we are making two assumptions: (1) that the effect of the quantitative matching variable is a smooth function of the variable, and (2) the sampling fractions vary smoothly with the matching variable. Both of these assumptions would in most cases seem reasonable, the first on purely biological grounds, the second because matching on a quantitative variable will always involve some (small) interval within which matching takes place, and so the strata of the population eligible (the basis for the sampling fractions) will tend to be overlapping for cases with similar values of the matching variable, which will lead to smoothly varying sampling fractions. At least this will be the case if the population distribution of the (quantitative) matching variable(s) is well behaved.

7.6 Nested case-control studies

The traditional way of phrasing the logic behind a case-control study is that controls should be representative for some background population. The assumption is that the relevant exposure or covariate information can be collected after cases and controls have been identified.

If a (large) population survey have been conducted where information on participants have been gathered—be that in the form of questionnaire answers, other forms of recordings, or biological samples—it may be prohibitively costly to extract exposure information from all participants in the survey. If a machinery for identifying cases of a disease of interest exists, a case-control study can be conducted among the participants in the survey.

The advantage is precisely as for a population-based case-control study: cost saving by only extracting the information needed for the cases and a set of controls, representing the follow-up time.

Often this is termed 'case-control study nested within a cohort', where the cohort refers to the follow-up of the initial sample with respect to disease outcome of interest.

In the Epi package there is a function ccwc (case-control within a cohort) that finds controls to cases recorded in a cohort. As a simple illustrative example we use the diet data from the Epi package. In order to match controls to cases we must specify when cases occur (case indicator fail (0/1), and the date of this exit), when persons are at risk (from entry to exit), and what time-scale we want the sampling to refer to (origin, assumed to be on the same scale as entry and exit):

```
> data( diet )
> set.seed( 1952 ) # random numbers will be reproducible
> ncc <- ccwc( entry = doe,
+                 exit = dox,
+                 fail = chd,
+               origin = dob,
```

```
+              controls = 2,
+                 match = job,
+               include = list(dob,doe,dox,energy),
+                  data = diet,
+                silent = FALSE )
Sampling risk sets: ...................................
> head( ncc )
  Set Map       Time Fail      job       dob       doe       dox
1   1   3 1984-03-20    1 Conductor 1919-12-24 1970-03-17 1984-03-20
2   1 191 1977-01-28    0 Conductor 1912-11-02 1972-08-16 1982-11-02
3   1 224 1980-01-11    0 Conductor 1915-10-16 1972-07-16 1985-10-15
4   2   9 1976-07-27    1 Conductor 1925-01-31 1971-03-17 1976-07-27
5   2 308 1976-03-27    0 Conductor 1924-10-01 1970-04-17 1986-12-02
6   2  82 1978-02-23    0 Conductor 1926-08-30 1969-09-16 1986-12-02
   energy
1 24.9537
2 25.6451
3 26.3510
4 23.1603
5 37.6690
6 25.9227
```

CODE EXPLAINED: After loading the data, we set the random number generator seed by set.seed, which makes the random numbers used by ccwc reproducible (otherwise, we would get a slightly different study every time we used ccwc). We want to match 2 controls (controls=2) to each case within the job category (match=job), choosing controls to each case among persons that are alive at the same *age* as the case. So we need to specify the time-scale origin as date of birth (origin=dob). Using head to list the first few lines of the resulting case-control data.

As noted in the beginning of this chapter, the controls should be chosen so they are representative of the risk time ('person-years') in the cohort. Therefore, there are no restrictions on the number of times a person can be included as control, and cases can even be included as controls as long as the index time is before the time of event (becoming a case).

In our example there are persons in the constructed case-control study that appear more than once:

```
> table( tt <- table(ncc$Map) )

  1   2   3
101  14   3
> who <- names( tt[tt>1] )
> with( subset(ncc, Map %in% who), table(Fail, Map) )
    Map
Fail 2 40 51 75 80 87 101 106 121 123 132 148 183 189 209 283 334
   0 3  2  1  2  2  2   2   3   1   2   2   1   1   1   2   1   2
   1 0  0  1  0  0  0   0   0   0   1   0   1   1   1   0   1   0
> ( wh.sets <- subset(ncc, Map %in% c(40,51))$Set )
[1]   3   6  25  26
> subset( ncc, Set %in% wh.sets )[,1:8]
  Set Map       Time Fail      job       dob       doe       dox
7   3  14 1973-03-28    1 Conductor 1912-08-08 1969-01-16 1973-03-28
8   3 253 1982-07-07    0 Conductor 1921-11-17 1970-07-17 1986-12-02
9   3  51 1978-02-01    0 Conductor 1917-06-14 1974-11-17 1979-07-01
```

```
16    6   51 1979-07-01    1 Conductor 1917-06-14 1974-11-17 1979-07-01
17    6  212 1974-10-17    0 Conductor 1912-09-30 1973-06-16 1982-09-30
18    6  101 1975-03-18    0 Conductor 1913-03-01 1973-04-16 1983-03-01
73   25  219 1969-08-31    1    Driver 1906-12-30 1969-01-16 1969-08-31
74   25    2 1975-03-07    0    Driver 1912-07-05 1973-07-16 1982-07-05
75   25   40 1983-03-21    0    Driver 1920-07-19 1969-03-16 1986-12-02
76   26  292 1986-05-07    1    Driver 1935-01-10 1971-06-17 1986-05-07
77   26   40 1971-11-14    0    Driver 1920-07-19 1969-03-16 1986-12-02
78   26   88 1974-06-20    0    Driver 1923-02-23 1970-11-17 1986-12-02
```

CODE EXPLAINED: The `table(ncc$map)` generates a table classified by `Map`, which is the persons' id, each entry being the number of times a person appears in the dataset `ncc`. Making a table of these table entries shows that there are 101 persons who appear once, 14 persons who appear twice, and 3 that appear three times. The vector `who` will contain the id of the persons that appear more than once. We then look at all persons in `ncc` that appear more than once (`subset(ncc,Map %in% who)`) and make a table of whether they appear as case or control. We see that person 40 appears as control twice, and person 51 once as case and once as control. We then find those matched sets where persons 40 and 51 appear.

Finally, we list all cases and controls selected to these matched sets—note the `%in%` operator; it selects those records from `ncc` where the value of `Set` is among the values in `wh.sets`.

We see that person 51 appears in set 6 as a case, with CHD at 1979-07-01 at age 62. The `Time` for the two matched controls is the date where they attain the same age as the case at the date of CHD. Person 51 also appear as control in set 3 at 1978-02-01, where he is the same age as the case, no. 14, 60 years.

Note that in the analysis of data the person included twice must be included with covariates corresponding to the index date (`Time`), so as a case in set 6 person 51 has age 62, but as control in set 3 he has age 60.

Analysis of nested case-control studies are precisely as the analysis of any other matched case-control study. In the example we used age as the time-scale for selection of controls, so the study is effectively matched on age (at event), and this variable should therefore be included in the models fitted. Since the matching is on a quantitative variable there is no need to do a conditional logistic regression; the matching variable (age in this case) can just be included in the model with a smooth effect.

But note that the `Time` variable in the resulting data frame is on the same scale as `entry` and `exit`, chosen as calendar time.

We might have used the explicitly computed age in the matching instead:

```
> set.seed( 1952 ) # random numbers will be reproducible
> diet <- transform( diet, aoe = (doe-dob)/365.25,
+                           aox = (dox-dob)/365.25 )
> acc <- ccwc( entry = aoe,
+               exit = aox,
+               fail = chd,
+             origin = 0,
+           controls = 2,
+              match = job,
+            include = list(dob,doe,dox,energy),
```

```
+                    data = diet,
+                  silent = FALSE )
Sampling risk sets: .........................................
> head( acc )
  Set Map    Time Fail       job        dob        doe        dox energy
1   1   3 64.23819    1 Conductor 1919-12-24 1970-03-17 1984-03-20 24.9537
2   1 191 64.23819    0 Conductor 1912-11-02 1972-08-16 1982-11-02 25.6451
3   1 224 64.23819    0 Conductor 1915-10-16 1972-07-16 1985-10-15 26.3510
4   2   9 51.48528    1 Conductor 1925-01-31 1971-03-17 1976-07-27 23.1603
5   2 308 51.48528    0 Conductor 1924-10-01 1970-04-17 1986-12-02 37.6690
6   2  82 51.48528    0 Conductor 1926-08-30 1969-09-16 1986-12-02 25.9227
```

> CODE EXPLAINED: The `transform` function allows for the creation of a new variable in a data frame; since `dob`, `doe`, and `dox` are date variables, the default unit of differences between them is days, so we scale the ages to years. We could have omitted `origin` since the default is 0. We see that the `Time` variable now is on the age scale, and that the age for all persons in each matched set is the same; it is the failure time for the case and the age at which covariates for the controls should be evaluated, which might be the number of prior hospitalizations. There are no such variables in this dataset, though.

7.6.1 *Register-based case-control studies*

With the advent of large registers of patients it is possible to follow patients, and occasionally entire populations (notably in the Nordic countries and Scotland) with respect to a particular disease occurrence. This gives the opportunity to describe absolute occurrence rates in the (patient) population. Occasionally these registers are used to derive case-control studies—essentially case-control studies nested in the register population. If no extra information is collected on cases and controls, there is no cost-saving involved relative to conducting a cohort study on the entire register. But the handling of data becomes easier because the datasets will be smaller.

However, this comes at the price of not being able to assess either the absolute occurrence rates or the effect of the chosen matching scale, be that age, calendar time, or date of birth. Recall from earlier that the matching variable must be included in the model, but that the estimated effect is the joint effect of the matching variable and the variation in the sampling fractions, and therefore not interpretable.

Thus, do not take the examples used here to illustrate the effects of nesting a case-control study in a cohort as representative of what should be done in real life. If you use `ccwc` to select controls in a cohort, you would normally want to collect some extra data on the cases and controls. If you already have all the data, there is no need to do a case-control study; you can just use the entire cohort and analyse the rates and rate ratios from that.

7.7 Case-cohort studies

As mentioned earlier, the rationale for a nested case-control study is often that data from a large population survey needs to be analysed without an excessive waste of resources. But a nested case-control study is designed to accommodate an estimation of effects on *one* specific outcome—controls are selected to match cases of one specific type.

If several outcomes are considered and the same covariates were of interest for these, say different cancers and/or types of CVD diagnoses, we could of course design a number of separate nested case-control studies, one for each type of outcome.

But intuitively it seems a bit wasteful; there ought to be a way to use the same controls to different types of outcome, instead of having a fresh set of controls for each type of case. And indeed there is, the case-cohort study design. While at first glance it looks like a variant of the case-control study, it really is a sophisticated sampling plan in a follow-up (survival) study, aimed at reducing data collection costs and yet obtaining almost the same precision as if we were using the entire cohort follow-up. Of course one could argue that so is a case-control study.

The idea is to select a random sub-cohort from the original cohort, at the time of entry (start of follow-up). Upon follow-up there will of course be some cases of the outcomes of interest in the sub-cohort. But since it is a sub-cohort the number of cases is most likely small, so not much information is available. But if we amend with the outcomes (cases, events) occurring *outside* of the cohort we can maximize the information.

The data collection costs amount to costs for the sub-cohort *plus* the costs for the cases that occur outside the sub-cohort. This is the key to use the design to assess the effect of covariates on several outcomes: the sub-cohort is the same for all types of outcome considered; the extra cost incurred by looking at a different outcome is the data collection costs for the different types of cases occurring outside the sub-cohort.

The analysis must of course take the sampling scheme into account; essentially, what is done is that the persons in the sub-cohort are entered as in an ordinary survival study, but the cases occurring *outside* the cohort enter follow-up immediately prior to the disease diagnosis, that is, with minimal follow-up time. A modified survival analysis is then made in order to produce estimates with the correct standard errors; there are a number of different approaches to the latter. These are implemented in the cch function from the survival package, here illustrated using the data from the National Wilm's Tumor Study available in the survival package:

```
> library( survival )
> data( nwtco )
> str( nwtco )
'data.frame':    4028 obs. of   9 variables:
 $ seqno       : int  1 2 3 4 5 6 7 8 9 10 ...
 $ instit      : int  2 1 2 2 2 1 1 1 1 2 ...
 $ histol      : int  2 1 2 1 2 1 1 1 1 1 ...
 $ stage       : int  1 2 1 4 2 2 4 2 1 2 ...
 $ study       : int  3 3 3 3 3 3 3 3 3 3 ...
 $ rel         : int  0 0 0 0 0 0 1 0 0 0 ...
 $ edrel       : int  6075 4121 6069 6200 1244 2932 324 5408 5215 1381 ...
 $ age         : int  25 50 9 28 55 32 45 44 123 31 ...
 $ in.subcohort: logi  FALSE FALSE FALSE TRUE FALSE FALSE ...

> nwtco <- transform( nwtco,
+                     histol = factor(histol, labels=c("FH","UH")),
+                     stage = factor(stage, labels=c("I","II","III","IV")),
+                     age = age / 12 )
> ccoh <- subset( nwtco, in.subcohort==1 | rel==1 )
> c( nrow(nwtco), nrow(ccoh) )
```

```
[1] 4028 1154
> with( ccoh, table(in.subcohort,rel) )
            rel
in.subcohort   0    1
      FALSE    0  486
       TRUE  583   85
```

> CODE EXPLAINED: The `transform` just puts sensible names on the levels of the categorical variables `histol` and `stage` by making them factors, and scales the age to years instead of months—for comparison purposes this is done in the entire original cohort. The `subset` function selects those who are in the chosen sub-cohort or who had an event (relapse)—some meet both criteria as seen from the table (`with` makes the `table` refer to variables in the `ccoh` data frame); there were 85 relapses in the sub-cohort and 486 outside. The `nrow` function simply counts the rows in the datasets, so we see that the case-cohort dataset has about a quarter of the records as the original dataset.

With these two datasets we con now compare the two analyses:

```
> fit.all <- coxph( Surv(edrel,rel) ~ stage + histol + age, data = nwtco )
> fit.ccp <-    cch( Surv(edrel,rel) ~ stage + histol + age, data = ccoh,
+                  subcoh = ~ in.subcohort,
+                      id = ~ seqno,
+             cohort.size = nrow(nwtco) )
```

> CODE EXPLAINED: We have the entire cohort so we can do a traditional survival analysis based on all available data, using `coxph` with time since diagnosis as the underlying time-scale, relapse of tumour as outcome and age (supplied in a `Surv` object), and stage and histology as explanatory variables.
>
> The case-cohort analysis using `cch` looks pretty much the same as the survival analysis, but we must additionally specify which of the persons were from the sub-cohort and which were cases occurring outside (`subcoh` argument), a person identifier (`id` argument)—both as a one-sided formula. Finally, we must also specify the size of the original cohort (`cohort.size` argument); the latter is necessary to get a handle on the absolute size of the rates.

We may compare the estimates obtained from the total database with those from the case-cohort sample, either by inspecting tables of estimates or more conveniently graphically:

```
> round( cbind( ci.exp(fit.all), ci.exp(fit.ccp) ), 3 )
         exp(Est.)  2.5% 97.5% exp(Est.)  2.5% 97.5%
stageII      1.949 1.536 2.473     2.085 1.498 2.900
stageIII     2.265 1.787 2.869     1.817 1.293 2.552
stageIV      3.170 2.434 4.129     3.991 2.672 5.963
histolUH     4.874 4.096 5.799     4.473 3.271 6.117
age          1.070 1.039 1.102     1.044 0.997 1.094
> plotEst( ci.exp(fit.ccp), xlog=TRUE, lwd=3, grid=c(5:9/10,1:10),
+             vref=1, xlab="Rate ratio" )
> linesEst( ci.exp(fit.all), y=5:1-0.2, col=gray(0.5), lwd=3 )
```

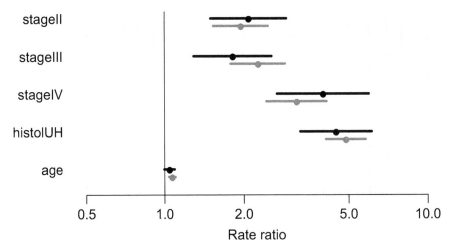

Figure 7.4 Forest plot of effect estimates for relapse hazard in the National Wilms Tumor Study. The black bars are from the case-cohort analysis; the grey bars are from the Cox-model for the entire dataset. RRs are relative to stage I, histology FH, and per 1 year of age.

CODE EXPLAINED: The function `ci.exp` returns the exponential of the estimated parameter with confidence intervals, while `cbind` just puts the two sets of estimates side by side. The function `plotEst` produces a so-called forest plot (Figure 7.4) of the estimates and confidence intervals from the case-cohort analysis, and `linesEst` adds the estimates from the Cox-model in grey colour.

Figure 7.4 shows that the estimates from the entire study and the case-cohort analysis are largely the same, but not surprisingly that the estimates from the total dataset have narrower confidence intervals. Note that the median age in the study is 3 years, so a scale for age in years *is* actually sensible; age just has a very small effect on relapse rates.

In summary, a case-cohort study is just a survival analysis based on a smartly chosen subset of data using a modified analysis method.

CHAPTER 8

Survival analysis

8.1 Introduction

Survival analysis concerns data where the outcome is a length of time, namely the time from inclusion in the study (such as diagnosis of some disease) till death or some other event—hence the term 'time to event analysis', which is also used. There are two primary targets normally addressed in survival analysis:

- Survival probabilities—the survival function:

$$S(t) = \mathrm{P}\{\text{Alive at } t \text{ after entry}\}$$

  Formally speaking, this is 1 – the cumulative distribution function of the survival time.
- Event rates—the probability of dying in the next small time interval, relative to the length of the interval:

$$\lambda(t) = \mathrm{P}\{\text{Death in } (t, t + \mathrm{d}t] | \text{ alive at } t\} / \mathrm{d}t$$

  Formally, the rate is the limit of this as $\mathrm{d}t \to 0$. A rate is also termed an intensity or a hazard.

The problem in using the survival function is that the observed survival times usually are *right censored*, which means that for some persons we do not know the survival time (life length), T, only that a person is still alive at some time c, the censoring time. So what we know is only that $T > c$ (assuming that everyone will eventually die).

This problem does not appear when we look at rates; the rate is only concerned with what happens just at some time t. Persons who die before t are disregarded, and persons' future history beyond t is not of relevance either—the rate is only concerned with what happens just around time t. The difference from survival is that the rate does not refer to an origin (entry time), but only to a point on the time-scale. As we shall see, focusing on rates also facilitates modelling, but at the expense of more elaborate data processing and extra work in derivation of measures that refer to some chosen origin.

As a very crude statement you can say that there is a one-to-one correspondence between the rates *plus* an origin, on one the hand, and the survival function, on the other.

8.2 Life table estimator of survival function

Before the advent of computers, estimation was based on tabulation in fairly crude intervals, say 1-year or 3-month intervals of time since entry. For each time interval the following is enumerated:

Epidemiology with R. Bendix Carstensen, Oxford University Press (2021). © Bendix Carstensen.
DOI: 10.1093/oso/9780198841326.003.0009

N number alive at the start of the interval

D number who died during the interval

L number who were censored / lost to follow-up during the interval.

The life table estimator computes the probability, π, of dying in an interval; a first shot could be $\hat{\pi} = D/N$, but that would *under*estimate the probability, because those censored were counted as if they were at risk of dying during the entire interval. But they might have died *after* they were censored and we should account for these (unknown) deaths. If we assume that the censored persons on average were removed halfway through the interval, the number of deaths they contribute during the half of the interval where their status is unknown is on average $L\pi/2$, so we should instead use

$$\pi = \frac{D + L\pi/2}{N} \quad \Rightarrow \quad \pi = \frac{D}{N - L/2}$$

This is known as the life table estimator of death probabilities.

The survival function is computed from these as the cumulative probability of surviving the intervals:

$$S(t_j) = P\{\text{survive interval } j \mid \text{entry to the first}\} = \prod_{i=1}^{i=j}(1 - \pi_i)$$

This is called the *life table* or *actuarial* estimator of the survival function.

Another approach is to compute the mortality *rate* in each interval using an assumption of censorings and deaths occurring halfway through the interval; so if the interval has length ℓ, the person-time in the interval is $(N - L/2 - D/2)\ell$ (assuming that deaths and censorings on average occur at the middle of the interval), then the mortality rate is $\lambda = D/((N - L/2 - D/2)\ell)$. The *cumulative* rate over the interval is therefore $\lambda\ell = D/(N - L/2 - D/2)$, and hence the survival probability is (Eq. (5.1), p. 96):

$$\pi = \exp\left(-D/(N - L/2 - D/2)\right)$$

The survival function based on this is called the *modified* life table estimator.

We can illustrate these estimators using the `lung` cancer survival data from the *survival* package; first, we load the relevant packages and the data (remember to do `?lung` to find out about the data):

```
> library( Epi )
> library( popEpi )
> library( survival )
> data( lung )
```

Then we make a table of censorings (`status=1`) and deaths (`status=2`) in 3-month intervals:

```
> lt <- with( lung, addmargins(
+                 table( cut(time/30,seq(0,36,3)),
+                     factor(status,labels=c("Alive","Dead"))) ) )
> head( lt, 3 )
        Alive Dead Sum
  (0,3]     0   27  27
  (3,6]     6   36  42
  (6,9]    22   30  52
> tail( lt, 3 )
```

```
           Alive Dead Sum
  (30,33]      1    0    1
  (33,36]      2    0    2
  Sum         63  165  228
> last <- nrow(lt)
> lt[,3] <- nrow(lung) - c(0,cumsum(lt[1:(last-1),3]))
> N <- lt[-last,3]
> D <- lt[-last,2]
> L <- lt[-last,1]
> cbind(N,D,L)

             N   D   L
(0,3]      228  27   0
(3,6]      201  36   6
(6,9]      159  30  22
(9,12]     107  24  13
(12,15]     70  16   7
(15,18]     47  10   4
(18,21]     33   7   4
(21,24]     22   8   0
(24,27]     14   5   2
(27,30]      7   2   2
(30,33]      3   0   1
(33,36]      2   0   2
```

CODE EXPLAINED: The cut function groups time (which we convert from days to months) in 3-month intervals from 0 to 36 months. Events and censorings (status) are then classified in these intervals by table. addmargins adds margins to the table, so that the third column of the table contains the total number of persons exiting (dead or censored) in each interval.

nrow tells how many rows there are in the table, so that we can refer to the last row with the total. If we take the total number of persons (which is in row last=nrow(lt)) and subtract the cumulative number of persons (cumsum) who die or are censored in each interval, we get the number at risk at the start of each interval. Thus lt now contains the numbers we need to compute the life table estimator, namely N, D, and L. For clarity of exposition we put them in three variables, N, D, and L, which we print side by side.

With this as a base, the formulae for the life table estimators derived above can be directly translated into code:

```
> pi <- D/(N-L/2)
> nn <- length(D)
> aS <- cumprod( c(1,1-pi[-nn]) )
> lm <- D/(N-L/2-D/2)
> mS <- cumprod( c(1,exp(-lm[-nn])) )
> round( cbind( N, D, L, pi, aS, mS ), 3 )
             N   D   L    pi    aS    mS
(0,3]      228  27   0 0.118 1.000 1.000
(3,6]      201  36   6 0.182 0.882 0.882
(6,9]      159  30  22 0.203 0.721 0.722
(9,12]     107  24  13 0.239 0.575 0.576
```

```
(12,15]  70  16   7  0.241  0.438  0.439
(15,18]  47  10   4  0.222  0.332  0.334
(18,21]  33   7   4  0.226  0.259  0.260
(21,24]  22   8   0  0.364  0.200  0.202
(24,27]  14   5   2  0.385  0.127  0.129
(27,30]   7   2   2  0.333  0.078  0.080
(30,33]   3   0   1  0.000  0.052  0.054
(33,36]   2   0   2  0.000  0.052  0.054
```

> CODE EXPLAINED: `pi` is computed as the actuarial estimator of the death probability in
> each interval; `cumprod` returns the cumulative product of its argument, that is, (1) the
> first element, (2) the product of the two first elements, (3) the product of the three first
> elements, etc. Doing this for the survival probabilities `1-pi` gives the survival function.
> But we must start with a 1, and so must omit the last element of `pi`, which is done by
> the index `-nn` (where `nn` is the length of the vectors); negative indexes *omit* elements
> from a vector
>
> The same is done for the modified life table estimator where the survival probability
> is `exp(-lm)`.

In practice there is no difference between the results from the two approaches as you see
from the print above and in Figure 8.1—unless of course data are *very* sparse.

There are of course formulae around to compute confidence limits for the survival
probabilities, but because the life table estimators are merely included for historical reasons
we shall not go there.

8.3 Kaplan–Meier estimator of survival

If we replace the 3-month intervals used in the actuarial estimator with increasingly
smaller intervals we will ultimately end with intervals that have at most 1 death or
censoring in each (and an awful lot of intervals with none). The estimate of the death
probability in an interval with 1 death and N persons at risk is $1/N$, and the survival
probability $(N - 1)/N$. The idea is therefore to leave the survival function constant
(horizontal) between death times, and at each death time decrease it by a factor $(N - 1)/N$.
This is the Kaplan–Meier estimator. Note that nothing happens at times where a censoring
occur.

If two deaths occur at the same time we can imagine that they occur a tiny bit apart,
so the change in survival probability at the first would be $(N - 1)/N$ and at the second
$(N - 2)/(N - 1)$. The product of these two is $(N - 2)/N$, which generalizes to $(N - k)/N$ if k
deaths are recorded at the same time. There is a number of other ways of handling survival
times recorded as identical, so-called *ties*. None of these make any big difference, so in
practice you can safely ignore choices of methods for handling ties; whatever the default
is, it has very little effect. Unless of course you have a very small dataset, in which case
you do not have much information about anything at all, and so it will not matter either.

Calculation of the Kaplan–Meier estimator is implemented in the `survfit` function in
the `survival` package:

```
> km0 <- survfit( Surv(time,status) ~ 1, data=lung )
> km0
```

```
Call: survfit(formula = Surv(time, status) ~ 1, data = lung)

    n  events  median 0.95LCL 0.95UCL
  228     165     310     285     363
```

> **CODE EXPLAINED:** The function `Surv` defines follow-up on a single time-scale, in this case starting at 0 ending at `time`, with censorings indicated by the smallest value of `status` (in this case 1, because `status` takes values 1 and 2). Because the r.h.s. of '~' is a `1`, `survfit` computes the Kaplan–Meier estimator for the entire dataset—and returns it in a `survfit` object, which we call km0.

We see that the default print method for a simple `survfit` object gives the total number of persons and deaths, as well as the median survival and a confidence interval for this. The median survival time is the time it takes for half of the initial population to die; it is a common summary measure of survival in a group of persons.

```
> plot( km0, yaxs = "i", xlab="Time since dagnosis (days)",
+                      ylab="Survival probability" )
> medsurv <- summary(km0)$table[7:9]
> abline( h=0.5 )
> points( medsurv, rep(0.5,3) )
> # add the actuarial estimators from above
> matlines( seq(0, 33, 3)*30, cbind(aS, mS),
+          type = "l", col = c("gray", "black"),
+          lty = c("solid", "22"), lend = "butt", lwd = 3, ylim = c(0,1) )
> lines( km0, lwd=2, conf.int=FALSE )
```

> **CODE EXPLAINED:** The `plot` (really `plot.survfit`) function plots the estimated survival curve—in this case the Kaplan–Meier estimator. By default, the confidence limits are shown in the plot (if there is only one curve). The argument `yaxs="i"` requires that the *y*-axis is *not* expanded a small amount in either end, and so is precisely from 0 to 1, reflecting that we are plotting a quantity (the survival probability) that necessarily is in the interval [0,1].
>
> Printing the km0 object gives the median survival time, and a little searching (try to do: `names(km0)` and `names(summary(km0))`, and querying the components by using `str()`) reveals that we can find it with 95% CI in `summary(km0)$table`, so we can plot them on the horizontal line at 0.5, showing that the confidence interval is where the confidence intervals for the survival crosses 0.5.
>
> For the sake of illustration we also show the life table estimators in the same plot. The two curves are plotted together using `matlines`; note that we computed the actuarial estimators using months (30-day intervals), but the Kaplan–Meier plot is with time measured in days, so we rescale to days when plotting. Choosing the line types (`lty`) as `"solid"`, respectively `"22"` (2 pixels of ink, 2 pixels blank), makes it possible to see both curves where they overlap. The `lend="butt"` determines that the endpoints of the broken lines are not rounded.
>
> The actuarial curves are plotted on top of the Kaplan–Meier estimator, so in order get the latter on top we plot it again, now with a thick line, but without the confidence intervals.

From Figure 8.1 we see that (1) there is no detectable difference between the life table estimators, (2) there is no substantial difference in conclusions that can be drawn from

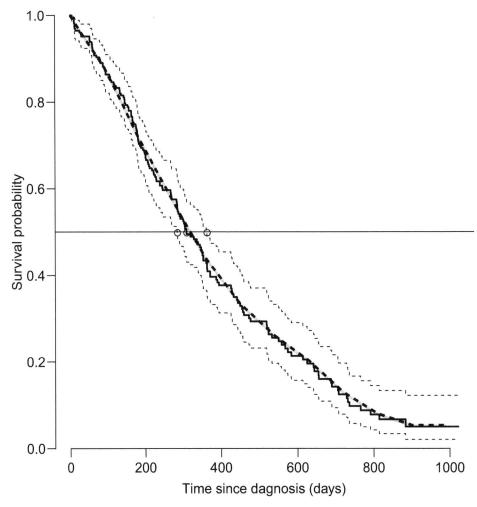

Figure 8.1 Kaplan–Meier estimator of survival after lung cancer with 95% CI (black) overlaid by the actuarial estimator (grey) and modified life table estimator (black, dotted).

the life table estimator and the Kaplan–Meier estimator (3) the Kaplan–Meier estimator looks like the life table estimator with random noise added.

8.3.1 *Survival in two groups*

We want to compare the survival of men and women. So we first convert `sex` to a factor in order to get human-readable output:

```
> lung <- transform( lung, sex = factor(sex,labels=c("M","W")) )
> plot( svsx <- survfit( Surv(time,status) ~ sex, data = lung ),
+       col=c("blue","red"), conf.int=TRUE, yaxs="i" )
> lines( svsx, col=c("blue","red"), lwd=2 )
> svsx
```

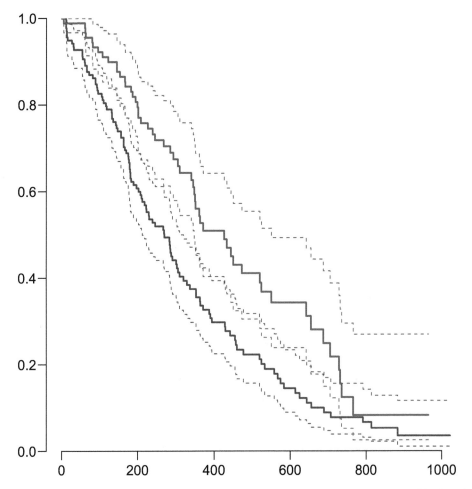

Figure 8.2 Kaplan–Meier estimates of survival after lung cancer by sex: men (blue) and women (red).

```
Call: survfit(formula = Surv(time, status) ~ sex, data = lung)

        n events median 0.95LCL 0.95UCL
sex=M 138    112    270     212     310
sex=W  90     53    426     348     550
```

CODE EXPLAINED: transform makes changes to a data frame, in this case lung, where sex is changed to a factor—the proper representation of a categorical variable.

When sex is placed on the r.h.s. of the formula in survfit, we get a Kaplan–Meier curve for each of the two sexes, and the plotting by default omits the confidence intervals, so we explicitly ask for these (conf.int=TRUE). The col argument gives the colours to be used for the two curves. Again we use yaxs="i" to ensure the *y*-axis is precisely from 0 to 1.

Note, we put the result of survfit in the object svsx, so we can plot the curves in the same plot with a slightly thicker line but without confidence intervals using lines.

If we want to test whether the survival for men and women is the same, we can compute the log-rank test (which we shall not derive here) using the `survdiff` function:

```
> survdiff( Surv(time,status) ~ sex, data = lung )
Call:
survdiff(formula = Surv(time, status) ~ sex, data = lung)

        N Observed Expected (O-E)^2/E (O-E)^2/V
sex=M 138      112     91.6      4.55      10.3
sex=W  90       53     73.4      5.68      10.3

 Chisq= 10.3  on 1 degrees of freedom, p= 0.001
```

So we see that there is a strongly significant difference in survival between men and women. In order to judge *how much* men and women differ we can refer to the graph of the two Kaplan–Meier curves, but we could also set up a model with some parameter to quantify the difference between men and women. By far the most widely used such model is the Cox model.

8.4 The Cox model

The Cox model is one for (mortality) *rates* that specifies the effect of covariates (such as sex) as log-linear and assumes that the effect is the same at any point on the time-scale:

$$\lambda(t, x_1, x_2, \ldots) = \lambda_0(t) \exp\left(\sum_j x_j \beta_j\right) = \lambda_0(t) \exp(\eta) \tag{8.1}$$

where $\eta = \sum_j x_j \beta_j$ is the *linear predictor*, providing a summary of the covariate effects.

Since the effect of the covariates is assumed to be the same over time, the ratio of the hazards for two persons with linear predictors η_1 and η_2 is

$$RR = \left((\lambda_0(t) \exp(\eta_1)\right) / \left((\lambda_0(t) \exp(\eta_2)\right) = \exp(\eta_1 - \eta_2)$$

which is independent of time. Since the ratio of the hazards is constant over time, we say that the hazards are proportional. This is why the Cox model often is called the proportional hazards model, although it is far from the only possible model with proportional hazards. If in the literature you come across the term 'proportional hazards model' as the only description of a model, It is a good bet that it refers to a Cox model, but also that it has been written hastily or by a person without strong statistical skills.

The model is fitted (that is, the βs are estimated) by maximizing Cox's *partial* (log-) likelihood:

$$\ell(\beta) = \sum_t \log\left(\frac{\exp(\eta_t)}{\sum_{i \in \mathcal{R}_t} \exp(\eta_i)}\right)$$

where the sum over t refers to all distinct death times, and $\mathcal{R}_t$ is the *risk set* at time t—the set of persons alive just before time t, including the person(s) that die at time t.

The practical estimation is by `coxph` (shorthand for cox proportional hazards model); note that the response must be a `Surv` object, usually created on the fly with the `Surv` function:

```
> c0 <- coxph( Surv(time,status) ~ sex + age, data = lung )
> summary(c0)
```

```
Call:
coxph(formula = Surv(time, status) ~ sex + age, data = lung)

  n= 228, number of events= 165

           coef exp(coef)  se(coef)       z Pr(>|z|)
sexW -0.513219  0.598566  0.167458  -3.065  0.00218
age   0.017045  1.017191  0.009223   1.848  0.06459

      exp(coef) exp(-coef) lower .95 upper .95
sexW     0.5986     1.6707    0.4311    0.8311
age      1.0172     0.9831    0.9990    1.0357

Concordance= 0.603  (se = 0.025 )
Likelihood ratio test= 14.12  on 2 df,   p=9e-04
Wald test              = 13.47  on 2 df,   p=0.001
Score (logrank) test = 13.72  on 2 df,    p=0.001
```

The interpretation is that women have a 40% smaller mortality after lung cancer than men of the same age (the W/M hazard ratio is 0.5986; see the column exp(coef)), while the mortality increases by 1.7% per year of age at diagnosis, for both men and women (the age estimate is 1.0172). It is assumed in the model that the *shape* of mortality as a function of time since diagnosis is the same for all persons, but there is nothing in the output that allows us to inspect this shape, i.e. how the mortality $\lambda_0(t)$ depends on time since diagnosis. So the effect of t (which is actually also a covariate) is bypassed in the estimation.

The simplest way to get a bit of a handle on how mortality depends on time is to plot the estimated survival function for specific values of the covariates, say a 60-year-old man and a 60-year-old woman:

```
> plot( survfit( c0, newdata = data.frame( sex = c("M","W"),
+                                           age = 60 ) ),
+       col = c("blue","red"), yaxs = "i", lwd = 2 )
```

CODE EXPLAINED: The newdata argument to survfit determines sets of covariates for which a survival curve is computed—you will get one survival curve for each row in newdata. The col argument puts different colours on the two resulting curves.

Note in Figure 8.3 that the two curves have jumps at exactly the same times as opposed to the two curves in Figure 8.2. The Kapan–Meier curves are estimated separately for men and women, without any assumptions about how the mortality rates for men and women are related. The estimates from the Cox model assume that mortality among men is 67% higher than among women at any time point, and this proportionality of rates translates into similar shapes of the survival curves (the log of the survival curves are proportional).

But even if the Cox model is formulated as a model for the mortality rates (λ) we cannot really get to see the rates (formally because they are not estimated in the modelling). The survival function is derived from what is normally called the Breslow estimator of the cumulative hazard; the rate itself is therefore the mathematical derivative of this. Since the Breslow estimator of the cumulative hazard is a step function, some effort is required to tease out the rate as the derivative of it—you may recall that a derivative requires a continuous function. Later we describe how to circumvent this problem (see section 8.6, p. 196 ff.).

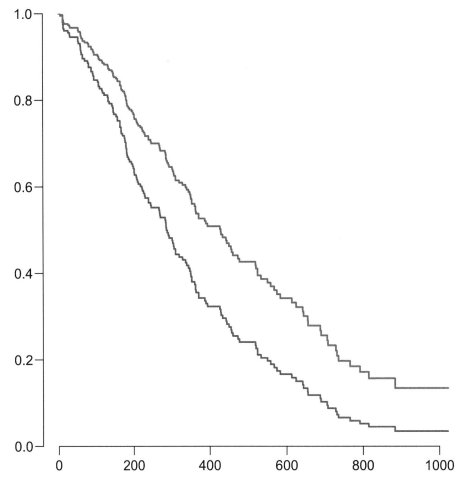

Figure 8.3 Estimated survival from a Cox model for men and women with lung cancer diagnosed at age 60.

8.4.1 *Mean survival or survival at mean?*

If we omit the `newdata` argument, `plot.survfit` will still produce a graph (which is not shown here):

```
> plot( prm0 <- survfit( c0 ) )
```

—the default behaviour is namely to use the mean of the covariates:

```
> with( lung, c( mean( as.numeric(sex) ), mean( age ) ) )
[1]   1.394737 62.447368
```

The resulting function is the survival function for a person aged 62.45 years with a sex of 1.395—39.5% woman and 60.5% man! Not very sensible. If you consult the help page of `survfit.coxph`, you will find a similar warning: 'since the resulting curve(s) almost never make sense'. Many other stats packages exhibit the same behaviour without a warning. Do not ever use `plot.survfit` without a `newdata` argument; it is most likely nonsense, but occasionally publishable in the clinical literature.

The resulting survival curve is *not* the expected survival of a group of patients with 39.5% women and 60.5% men and mean age 62.45. The latter is not well defined—even for given fixed effects of age and sex; the survival of a given group of patients depends on the entire distribution of age and sex, not only on the means of the two variables.

We can illustrate this by computing the expected survival curve for each of the persons in the lung dataset, and then take the mean of these survival curves. The result depends on the particular distribution of age in the dataset—and we can construct any number of different data sets with 39.5% women and mean age of 62.4 years. For illustration we use the lung dataset:

```
> nd.lung <- lung[,c("sex","age")]
> prlu <- survfit( c0, newdata=nd.lung )
> lusurv <- apply( prlu$surv, MARGIN=1, mean )
```

> CODE EXPLAINED: The fitted Cox model, c0, has two explanatory variables, sex and age, so if we want the expected survival we must supply a data frame (new data, hence the prefix nd) with variables age and sex, the former in years, the latter a factor with levels M and F. The first statement just selects the two variables from the lung data frame. If we supply this as newdate to survfit, it generates 228 survival curves, each consisting of the survival probability at 186 time points (corresponding to the different times in prlu$time), arranged in a 186 × 228 matrix, prlu$surv. apply calculates the mean over each row of the argument, so the result is a vector of length 186 (corresponding to MARGIN 1), with the average of the survival probabilities corresponding to the time-points in prlu$time (try str(prlu)). This is the expected survival of a population with an age and sex distribution as that of the lung data.

We also generate the mean survival in another population with the same mean age and the same percentage of women, but deliberately chosen to be very inhomogeneous:

```
> xnd.lung <- data.frame( sex = rep(c("W","M"),c(90,138)),
+                         age = rep(c(40,90),c(126,102)) )
> c( mean(lung$age), mean(xnd.lung$age) )

[1]  62.44737 62.36842

> xprlu <- survfit( c0, newdata = xnd.lung )
> xlusurv <- apply( xprlu$surv, MARGIN=1, mean )
```

> CODE EXPLAINED: The rep generates 90 copies of W and 138 of M (corresponding to the sex-distribution in lung), and also 126 copies of 40 and 102 copies of 90, which will produce (almost) the same mean age in the xnd.lung as in nd.lung.
> The expected survival for this population is calculated exactly as for nd.lung.

We now plot the survival curve for an average person (in grey), and the expected survival for the actual population in the data set, as well as the expected survival for an extremely inhomogeneous population:

```
> plot( prm0, conf.int = FALSE, col = gray(0.7), lwd = 2, yaxs = "i",
+       xlab = "Time since dagnosis (days)",
+       ylab = "Survival probability" )
> lines( prlu$time,  lusurv, type = "s", lwd = 1 )
> lines( xprlu$time, xlusurv,
+        type = "s", lty = "21", lend = "butt", lwd = 2 )
```

CODE EXPLAINED: The plot (really plot.survfit because prm0 has class survfit) plots the survival for a single person with sex equal to the mean sex (nonsense, remember?) and age equal to the mean age of persons in the lung data set with a grey line. lines plots the expected survival for the study population with a black line, using type="s" to get the steps. This is also used to plot the resulting expected survival curve for the inhomogeneous population with a broken line (lty="21": 2 pixels of ink, 1 pixel blank).

From Figure 8.4 we see that that the black curve—the curve is the one that makes properly probabilistic sense as the expected survival of the patient population—is a tiny bit below the grey one in the beginning and above it towards the end.

This is the selection phenomenon, also called the *frailty* phenomenon, which is even more pronounced for the broken curve with the very inhomogeneous population. In the

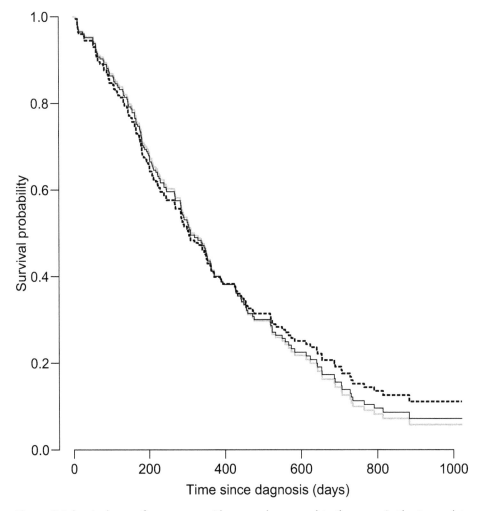

Figure 8.4 Survival curve for a person with age and sex equal to the mean in the lung data set, the default (grey), the mean of the expected survival curves for the persons in the dataset (black), and the mean of the survival curves for a population with very spread agedistribution (broken). All curves are based on the Cox model with sex and age as explanatory variables.

beginning the persons with high mortality (old men—the most frail) die first, so as time goes by, they are removed from the population at risk, and younger women will be relatively more prominent among those at risk. In contrast to this, the grey curve is computed as if the age and sex compositions were the same throughout the follow-up time (it is a survival curve for a group of identical—and quite funny—persons). So in the heterogeneous population the *overall* mortality is higher in the beginning and smaller towards the end. Which is reflected in the survival curves. This is seen in a more extreme form in the dotted curve for the very inhomogeneous population.

So briefly (and imprecisely): survival of an average person is different from the average survival of persons.

Therefore, when computing predicted survival curves:

- *Never* use the default behaviour; if you have categorical variables in the model you get sheer nonsense predictions. Even if you have only quantitative variables, who wants to see the expected survival of a person aged 62.45 years?—the age which just happens to be the mean age in *this* study.
- Remember that the estimated survival curve for *one* given set of covariates can be interpreted as the expected survival of a large group of *identical* persons—identical in terms of covariate values. As this group is decimated by death, the characteristics of the survivors' covariate distribution do not change.

  Alternatively it can be interpreted as a probability statement for a particular person—in the example above a woman aged 60 years at diagnosis. This is presumably what you want in most practical circumstances.
- If you compute the average survival of an inhomogeneous population the result depends on the *entire joint distribution* of covariates, not only on their means.

8.5 The time-scale

The lung cancer example we just used was not strictly speaking an epidemiological dataset, it was from clinical medicine; and it carries the central characteristic that all patients start at the same time, namely at lung cancer diagnosis. Without any discussion we just assumed that time since diagnosis was the relevant time-scale. This is a characteristic of clinical data: there is normally one clearly primary time-scale of interest.

Looking at the dataset `DMlate` from the `Epi` package consisting of follow-up of (a random sample of) diabetes patients from Denmark, we will describe how mortality depends on different time-scales, age, calendar time, and diabetes duration.

```
> library( Epi )
> library( popEpi )
> data( DMlate )
> head( DMlate )
       sex    dobth     dodm     dodth    dooad doins      dox
50185    F 1940.256 1998.917       NA       NA    NA 2009.997
307563   M 1939.218 2003.309       NA 2007.446    NA 2009.997
294104   F 1918.301 2004.552       NA       NA    NA 2009.997
336439   F 1965.225 2009.261       NA       NA    NA 2009.997
245651   M 1932.877 2008.653       NA       NA    NA 2009.997
216824   F 1927.870 2007.886 2009.923       NA    NA 2009.923
> DMlate <- subset( DMlate, dox > dodm )
```

If we use current age as the time-scale we have the problem that not all persons (in fact, none at all) start at the same time or age. In survival analysis, this phenomenon is called *delayed entry*, *staggered entry*, or *left truncation*. In epidemiology it's just a fact of life. It can be handled by Surv too, by adding an extra argument with the entry time as the first:

```
> aDM <- coxph( Surv(dodm-dobth, dox-dobth, !is.na(dodth)) ~ sex,
+               data=DMlate )
> dDM <- coxph( Surv(           dox-dodm , !is.na(dodth)) ~ sex,
+               data=DMlate )
> pDM <- coxph( Surv(dodm       , dox      , !is.na(dodth)) ~ sex,
+               data=DMlate )
> round( rbind( ci.exp(aDM), ci.exp(dDM), ci.exp(pDM) ), 3 )
      exp(Est.)  2.5% 97.5%
sexF      0.676 0.624 0.733
sexF      0.891 0.823 0.964
sexF      0.889 0.822 0.962
```

> CODE EXPLAINED: In the first use of coxph each person enters at the age of diabetes diagnosis (dodm-dobth), and exits at the age at exit (dox-dobth), a death outcome indicated by a non-missing date of death (!is.na(dodth)).
>
> In the second we are using time since diagnosis of diabetes as the time-scale, and in the third calendar time, but of course all with the same indicator of death. Since the start time on the duration time-scale is 0 for all persons, we can omit the first argument to Surv. To be perfectly aligned with the two other cases we could have written dodm-dodm as the entry time on the duration scale.
>
> At the end we use rbind to put the estimates of the sex-effects underneath each other, and finally we round them to three decimals with round.

We see that the estimated difference for mortality between men and women is large when we use age as the time-scale, and substantially smaller when using diabetes duration or calendar time. There is apparently a substantial confounding by current age in the two latter estimates. For now it suffices to note that choice of time-scale may influence effect estimates. In this respect, time-scales do not differ from any other potential confounders, and in particular it should be noted that there is no *external* way of deciding which time-scale to choose; choice of time-scale will always be an *empirical* question.

We can use the plot.survfit to show the survival curves:

```
> par( mfrow=c(1,3), yaxs="i" )
> plot( aa <- survfit( aDM, newdata=data.frame(sex=c("M","F")) ),
+       col=c("blue","red"), xlab="Current age", lwd=1, conf.int=TRUE )
> lines( aa, col=c("blue","red"), lwd=2 )
> plot( dd <- survfit( dDM, newdata=data.frame(sex=c("M","F")) ),
+       col=c("blue","red"), xlab="DM duration", lwd=1, conf.int=TRUE )
> lines( dd, col=c("blue","red"), lwd=2 )
> plot( pp <- survfit( pDM, newdata=data.frame(sex=c("M","F")) ),
+       col=c("blue","red"), xlab="Calendar time", lwd=1,
+       xlim=c(1990,2010), ylim=0:1, conf.int=TRUE )
> lines( pp, col=c("blue","red"), lwd=2 )
```

> CODE EXPLAINED: We set up a 1-by-3 layout of graphs by `par(mfrow=c(1,3))`, and plot the standard survival curves from the models with different time-scales. The default for `plot.survfit` is to start the survival curve at 0, which makes no sense for calendar time, so we have set the x-axis to a sensible range, namely where we actually have data.
>
> The curves are plotted with confidence intervals (`conf.int=TRUE`), and then the curve is plotted with a thicker line (`lwd=2`) for clarity.

If we use age as time-scale as in the leftmost panel of Figure 8.5, where persons enter after time 0 (called left truncation or staggered entry), it is difficult to assign a reasonable interpretation to the survival curves; formally, it would be survival from birth, but in the age range 0–20 we have almost no data, and it's absurd to have a curve that implicitly refers to the survival of a group of newborns with diabetes. The persons we are modelling do not get diabetes till later in life. Further more, we are using the assumption that the age-specific mortality rates do not depend on either duration or age at diagnosis. The uncertainty is very large because we have very sparse data for ages under 30, so any measure, such as the survival, cumulated from age 0 will carry a large uncertainty.

The middle panel in Figure 8.5 is easier to interpret; it is the survival for diabetes patients from date of diagnosis, assuming that neither age at diagnosis nor current age influences mortality. But the curves are based on data with substantial amounts of information in the early part of the time-scale. Hence the cumulative measure from duration 0 does not suffer from initial uncertainty.

The rightmost panel in Figure 8.5 is for a time period from 1990 onward because the time-scale is calendar time. It represents the survival since 1995 because this is from where we have data, but the curve by default stretches all the way to 0. The assumption is that the mortality of diabetes patients only depends on calendar time and not on age or duration.

The conclusion here is that you should only show survival curves when you have data with observation from some sensible time origin (often 0).

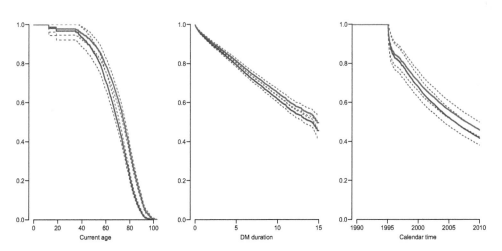

Figure 8.5 Estimated survival curves for Danish diabetes patients using different time-scales; men in blue, women in red.

But the fact that a survival curve along the age-axis is irrelevant does not mean that current age may not be a relevant covariate in the analysis of mortality rates. It is not the *model* that is goofy; it is the transformation to 'survival since birth' that is.

8.6 Relation between Cox and Poisson models

To illustrate the relationship between Cox and Poisson models we again use the `lung` dataset from the `survival` package; it has survival times for lung cancer patients, and you want to use '`?lung`' to remind yourself of the data.

In the definition of the Cox model in (8.1) the shape of the baseline hazard is left unspecified; the Cox model implicitly takes it as being as detailed as possible given the data, the cumulative rate having a jump at every event time. If we move to the other extreme and assume that the baseline hazard is constant over time it turns out that the likelihood for the survival data, *including* the single baseline rate as a parameter, is a Poisson likelihood (see section 5.2.2), which we can fit by the `poisreg` family:

```
> lung$sex <- factor( lung$sex, labels=c("M","W") )
> c0 <- coxph( Surv(time, status) ~ sex + age, data = lung )
> p0 <- glm( cbind(status==2, time) ~ sex + age,
+          family = poisreg, data = lung )
> round( cbind( ci.exp(c0), ci.exp(p0)[-1,] ), 3 )
     exp(Est.)  2.5% 97.5% exp(Est.)  2.5% 97.5%
sexW     0.599 0.431 0.831     0.618 0.446 0.858
age      1.017 0.999 1.036     1.016 0.998 1.034
```

> CODE EXPLAINED: The coxph just fits the Cox model with age and sex as covariates; the glm with family `poisreg` fits a Poisson model which has the same likelihood as a mortality model with constant rate. The Cox model `c0` only has the regression parameters for sex and age; the Poisson model also has an intercept which is omitted by the '`[-1,]`'. The intercept would correspond to the mortality for a man aged 0, in units of deaths per day (because the variable `time` is survival time in days)—not very sensible.

We can centre the age and scale the time in the Poisson model to get interpretable parameters:

```
> c0 <- coxph( Surv(time,status) ~ sex + I((age-60)/10), data = lung )
> p0 <- glm( cbind(status==2,time/365.25) ~ sex + I((age-60)/10),
+          family=poisreg, data = lung )
> round( cbind( rbind(NA,ci.exp(c0)), ci.exp(p0) ), 3 )
                   exp(Est.)  2.5% 97.5% exp(Est.)  2.5% 97.5%
                        NA    NA    NA     0.997 0.819 1.214
sexW                 0.599 0.431 0.831     0.618 0.446 0.858
I((age - 60)/10)     1.186 0.990 1.421     1.169 0.978 1.397
```

> CODE EXPLAINED: The risk time is now entered as `time/365.25`, which means that the estimated (constant) baseline rate (the intercept in the model) will appear in units of deaths per 1 year. We subtracted 60 from age which means that the intercept refers to the mortality rate among 60-year-old men. We also divided it by 10, which means that the age parameter now is the rate ratio between two persons with an age

difference of 10 years. Since '-' and '/' have special meaning in model formulae it is necessary to wrap any expression with these in the function 'I', which is just the identity function; I(x)=x for any x.

In order to print the estimates from the two models side by side with cbind, we must insert a row of NAs on top of the estimates from the Cox model to get a matrix with 3 rows that will match the one from the Poisson model.

We see that the estimates of effects of sex and age are quite similar between the two approaches: women have a mortality which is about 60% of that for men, and mortality increases about 17% per 10 years of age at diagnosis. Also the confidence intervals are pretty similar.

The (exponentiated) intercept parameter from the Poisson model is the overall mortality rate per 1 year for a 60-year-old man—it is around 1 per person-year—lung cancer is indeed a very lethal disease.

This is but an example and it is possible to find examples where the assumption of constant baseline mortality more strongly influences the parameter estimates. But as we shall see in the next section this can be remedied.

8.6.1 Simple parametric mortality functions

In section 5.5 we saw how to model mortality rates using assumptions about constant mortality rates in very small intervals and putting parametric restrictions on the *size* of the rates in each interval. If we do this for the mortality rates from lung cancer we can convert the estimated mortality rates to a survival function.

The requirement is that we split the follow-up in to small intervals, which is easiest if we set up the follow-up in a Lexis diagram:

```
> Ll <- Lexis( exit = list(tfd=time),
+         exit.status = factor(status,labels=c("Alive","Dead")),
+               data = lung )
NOTE: entry.status has been set to "Alive" for all.
NOTE: entry is assumed to be 0 on the tfd timescale.
> Sl <- splitMulti( Ll, tfd=seq(0,1200,20) )
> summary( Ll )
Transitions:
     To
From   Alive Dead  Records:  Events: Risk time:  Persons:
  Alive   63  165       228      165     69593        228
> summary( Sl )
Transitions:
     To
From   Alive Dead  Records:  Events: Risk time:  Persons:
  Alive 3432  165      3597      165     69593        228
> Sl[1:6+13,1:10]
   lex.id tfd lex.dur lex.Cst lex.Xst inst time status age sex
1:      1 260      20   Alive   Alive    3  306      2  74   M
2:      1 280      20   Alive   Alive    3  306      2  74   M
3:      1 300       6   Alive    Dead    3  306      2  74   M
4:      2   0      20   Alive   Alive    3  455      2  68   M
5:      2  20      20   Alive   Alive    3  455      2  68   M
6:      2  40      20   Alive   Alive    3  455      2  68   M
```

> CODE EXPLAINED: The `Lexis` function sets up a `Lexis` object with one time-scale, `tfd` (time from diagnosis), and exit status according to whether `status` takes value 1 or 2. Unlike the specification in section 5.3, we have omitted the `entry` specification which has a default of 0 for all persons—this is only possible if there is only *one* time-scale in the `Lexis` object. `splitMulti` subdivides the follow-up every 20 days, and `summary` shows the number of records in the split dataset. The last statement just lists the last few records of person (`lex.id`) 1 and the first few from person 2 from the split dataset illustrating the outcome variable `lex.Xst`.

We can model the mortality rates by a smooth function of the time at the start of each interval by using the `gam` function from the `mgcv` package. The `gam` function can be accessed through the wrapper and `gam.Lexis` designed to fit a Poisson model to data in a `Lexis` data frame:

```
> p0 <- gam.Lexis( Sl, formula = ~ s(tfd) + sex + I((age-60)/10) )
mgcv::gam Poisson analysis of Lexis object Sl with log link:
Rates for the transition: Alive->Dead
> round( cbind( ci.exp(c0), ci.exp(p0, subset=c("sex","age")) ), 3 )
                  exp(Est.)  2.5% 97.5% exp(Est.)  2.5% 97.5%
sexW                  0.599 0.431 0.831     0.603 0.435 0.837
I((age - 60)/10)      1.186 0.990 1.421     1.177 0.983 1.410
```

> CODE EXPLAINED: The `gam.Lexis` fits a Poisson model with penalized splines (`s()`) for the baseline (`tfd`) effect on mortality rates, a categorical effect of sex and a linear effect of age at diagnosis (`age`). `ci.exp` extracts the regression parameters from the Cox model `c0` and the Poisson model `p0`, and `cbind` lists them side by side.

The specification of the `gam` model is more logical than for the `Cox` model; the baseline time-scale (in this case `tfd`) is specified together with the other covariates.

We see that the estimates of the sex and age effects from the two models are very close; this will normally be the case if the effect of the time-scale is modelled reasonably flexibly.

Baseline mortality rate

The Poisson model has the advantage that we have an easily accessible estimate of the baseline `hazard`, in the Cox model termed $\lambda_0(t)$, but which is not directly available from the Cox model.

This requires that we specify values for *all* covariates in the model, including the time-scale, `tfd`. We compute baseline hazards for men and women aged 60, for times 0–1000 days after diagnosis:

```
> ndm <- data.frame( tfd=seq(0,1000,10), age=60, sex="M" )
> ndw <- data.frame( tfd=seq(0,1000,10), age=60, sex="W" )
> prm <- ci.pred( p0, ndm ) * 3650
> prw <- ci.pred( p0, ndw ) * 3650
> rr  <- ci.exp( p0, ctr.mat = list(ndm,ndw) )
> matshade( ndm$tfd, cbind( prm, prw ), plot=TRUE,
+          log="y", col=c(4,2), lwd=2, lty=1, ylim=c(0.5,50),
+          xlab="Time since diagnosis (days)",
+          ylab="Mortality rate per 10 PY / M/W Rate Ratio" )
> matshade( ndm$tfd, rr, lwd=2 )
> abline( h=1, lty=3 )
```

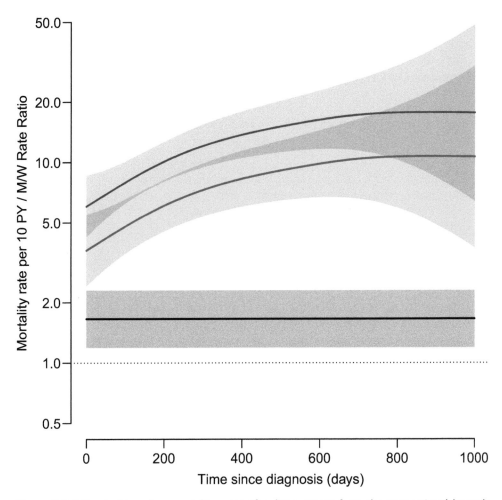

Figure 8.6 Estimated baseline mortality rates after lung cancer from the proportional hazards model. Men are in blue, women are in red, and the rate ratio is in black. The shaded areas correspond to 95% confidence intervals.

CODE EXPLAINED: We define two prediction data frames with times from 0 to 1000 days, one for men aged 60 and one for women aged 60. `ci.pred` will then compute mortality rates for these from the model `p0`, but in units of deaths per 1 day, so we multiply by 3650 to get it per 10 years. We also compute the rate ratio between men and women using the facility of `ci.exp` that when a `list` of two data frames is provided as the second argument, it will compute the rate ratio between predictions from the data frames.

The two sets of predictions—men and women—are then plotted with shaded confidence intervals, using `matshade`. Note that with the argument `plot=TRUE`, `matshade` will create new plot; without that it will add to an existing plot.

The rate ratio is then added to the plot using `matshade`. Finally, we add a horizontal line at RR=1.

The Poisson model p0 is a proportional hazards models, so the hazards for men and women are proportional; they have constant distance on a log-scale. From Figure 8.6 we see that the rate ratio is constant over time.

We also see that the baseline mortality is increasing steeply in the beginning and flattening after about a year.

Survival curves

In order to get the predicted survival curve from the model with the smoothly varying baseline hazard, we need a prediction data frame with one row per time point of prediction:

```
> nd <- data.frame( tfd=seq(0,1000,10)+5, sex="W", age=60 )
> sv.w <- ci.surv( p0, nd, int=10 )
> plot( survfit( c0, newdata = data.frame( sex="W",age=60)), yaxs="i" )
> matshade( nd$tfd-5, sv.w, col="red", lwd=2 )
```

CODE EXPLAINED: The prediction data frame nd is a data frame for the mortality predictions; predictions will be made at midpoints of intervals from 0 to 1000 days in steps of 10, for a 60-year-old woman. ci.surv computes the mortality rates for these covariate values and converts to the survival function, including the confidence intervals. In order to do this we must supply the length of the interval between the prediction points to ci.surv; it is a requirement that the prediction points (in nd$tfd) are equally spaced, in this case 10 days apart.

Note that there is no necessary relationship between the length of the intervals into which we split the follow-up (here, 20 days) and the intervals we use for calculating the survival curve (here, 10 days). The former need not even have the same length; the latter do.

The plot (i.e. plot.survfit) draws the estimated survival function for a 60-year-old woman based on the Cox model, with confidence limits as broken lines, and matshade overlays the plot with the estimated survival function from the model with smooth baseline hazard with confidence limits as shaded areas.

We may want to show the survival curves for 60-year-old men too; this is quite easily done:

```
> plot( survfit(c0, newdata = data.frame(sex=c("W","M"), age=60)),
+       conf.int=TRUE, col = c("red","blue"), yaxs = "i" )
> nd <- transform( nd,  sex = "M" )
> sv.m <- ci.surv( p0, nd, int = 10 )
> matshade( nd$tfd-5, cbind(sv.w,sv.m), col = c("red","blue"), lwd = 2 )
```

CODE EXPLAINED: survfit has the advantage that the points of prediction of the survival curve are just the event times and so need not be specified explicitly. This is not the case when using ci.surv for a parametric model. So with survfit the specification of two predicted survival curves just requires a two-line data frame, while prediction by ci.surv requires a an entire prediction frame with all time points for each new survival curve.

The prediction data frame is changed using transform so it refers to a man, and thus we can produce the survival curve for a 60-year-old man, and plot the two curves in the same plot. plot.survfit will plot two stepcurves (with confidence limits, conf.int=TRUE), and matshade plots the two parametric curves.

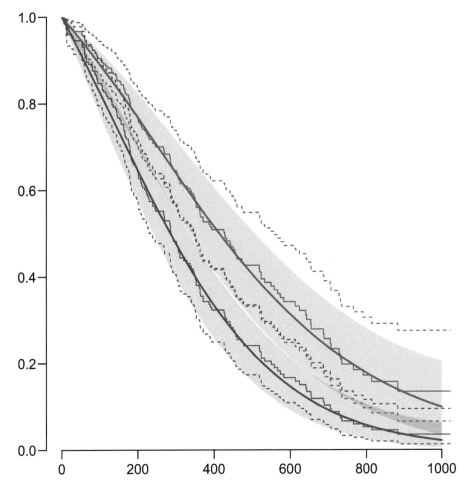

Figure 8.7 Survival curves for men (blue) and women (red) from a Cox model and a Poisson model with smooth underlying hazard. The step functions are the estimated survival curves from the Cox model, the thin lines indicating the 95% confidence intervals; the estimates from the Poisson model are full lines with 95% confidence intervals as shaded areas.

From Figure 8.7 we see that the two approaches produce substantially the same type of conclusions, but it is also clear that the curves from the parametric model are biologically far more credible than the stepcurves produced by the Cox model approach.

In summary, parametric survival curves can be obtained through the following steps: (1) Set up the follow-up data in a Lexis object, (2) fit a gam model using gam.Lexis, (3) set up a prediction data frame with the time points for the survival and any other covariates in the model, (4) use ci.surv to get the survival curve, and (5) plot it, e.g. with matshade.

A non-parametric curve is obtained through the following steps: (1) Set up the follow-up data in a Surv object, (2) fit a Cox model using coxph, (3) set up a prediction data frame with the values of the regression covariates in the model, (4) use survfit to get the survival curve, and (5) plot it, e.g. with plot (really plot.survfit).

8.6.2 *Proportional hazards?*

The main assumption in the Cox model is that of proportional hazards, in the lung cancer example that the rate ratio between men and women is constant as a function of time, and for the age variable that the rate ratio between any two ages will be constant as a function of time.

These hypotheses can be tested using `cox.zph` which provides a p-value of the hypothesis of proportionality against a model with interaction between the variable and the time variable. The function has a `plot` method, which will plot the Shoenfeld residuals versus time—if there are no deviations from proportional hazards, the average of these residuals should be constant across time:

```
> ( zz <- cox.zph( c0 ) )
                   chisq df    p
sex                2.608  1 0.11
I((age - 60)/10) 0.209  1 0.65
GLOBAL             2.771  2 0.25

> par( mfrow=c(1,2))
> plot( zz )
```

To the extent that the residuals' average vary over time, the variation indicates how the interaction between the covariate and time may look. Judging from Figure 8.8 there does not seem to be any meaningful age-by-time interaction, but it looks like there might be a monotone trend in the M/W rate ratio.

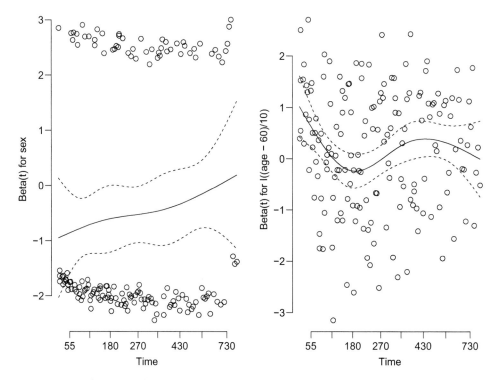

Figure 8.8 Default plot from `cox.zph`, showing Shoenfeld residuals versus time and the smoothed averages for each of the two covariates in the model.

However, if we are looking for an interaction, it would be more useful to estimate a proper interaction and inspect the shape of it in order to judge whether it is worth bothering about, regardless whether the p-value is a bit below or above 5%. This will also have the advantage that we can report the shape of it from a properly specified interaction model. Returning to the example, we would fit a model with time (tfd) interaction with sex:

```
> ps <- gam.Lexis( S1, formula = ~ s(tfd, by=sex) + sex + age )
mgcv::gam Poisson analysis of Lexis object S1 with log link:
Rates for the transition: Alive->Dead
> anova( ps, p0, test="Chisq")
Analysis of Deviance Table

Model 1: cbind(trt(Lx$lex.Cst, Lx$lex.Xst) %in% trnam, Lx$lex.dur) ~
  s(tfd, by = sex) + sex + age
Model 2: cbind(trt(Lx$lex.Cst, Lx$lex.Xst) %in% trnam, Lx$lex.dur) ~
  s(tfd) + sex + I((age - 60)/10)
  Resid. Df Resid. Dev      Df Deviance Pr(>Chi)
1    3590.9    1298.0
2    3591.4    1299.5 -0.52822  -1.4688   0.1092
```

> CODE EXPLAINED: The interaction is specified through the by= argument as a separate spline for each sex, but we must keep the main effect of sex in the model; otherwise, we would be defining a model where the mortality in men and women coincided at a specific time (roughly the middle for the time range).
>
> In the graph, it looks as if the log-mortality rate for women is a linear function of time since diagnosis. In fact it is only approximately so; from the model summary we see that the smooth term for women has effective degrees for freedom (edf) very close to 1, meaning that the curve has been penalized to be (almost) linear.
>
> The anova function compares the two models using a log-likelihood ratio test (test="Chisq").

We see that there is not much improvement in deviance by adding an interaction (p-value 0.11), but we plot the rates and the M/W rate ratio from the estimated interaction model to inspect the shape of the interaction:

```
> ndm <- data.frame( tfd=seq(0,1000,10), age=60, sex="M" )
> ndw <- data.frame( tfd=seq(0,1000,10), age=60, sex="W" )
> prm <- ci.pred( ps, ndm ) * 3650
> prw <- ci.pred( ps, ndw ) * 3650
> rr  <- ci.exp( ps, ctr.mat = list(ndm,ndw) )
> matshade( ndm$tfd, cbind( prm, prw ), plot=TRUE,
+          log="y", col=c(4,2), lwd=2, lty=1, ylim=c(0.5,50),
+          xlab="Time since diagnosis (days)",
+          ylab="Mortality rate per 10 PY / M/W Rate Ratio" )
> matshade( ndm$tfd, rr, lwd=2 )
> abline( h=1, lty=3 )
```

> CODE EXPLAINED: This bit of code is almost identical to that used earlier (p. 198) when showing the baseline hazards, the only difference being the model from which the predictions are made, ps instead of p0.

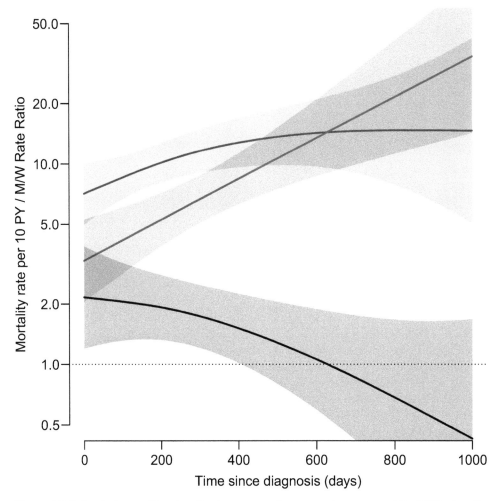

Figure 8.9 Estimated mortality rates after lung cancer for men and women and the M/W rate ratio. Men are in blue, women are in red, and the rate ratio is in black. The shaded areas correspond to 95% confidence intervals.

From Figure 8.9 we see that despite the p-value for interaction between sex and time there is a clear indication that men mainly have a higher mortality than women during the first year or so after diagnosis of lung cancer. So despite a p-value of about 10% there actually *is* some interaction of interest.

Occasionally it is seen that a significant test from cox.zph is followed by separate analyses for an early and a late period of the time-scale. This corresponds to a very simplistic interaction, based on a dichotomization of a quantitative variable in interaction with a quantitative time effect. This will carry the same problems as any other dichotomization of a quantitative variable, and should be avoided; see Chapter 9.

So the proportionality of hazards is not a question of testing; it is a question of evaluating an interaction with the time-scale in the light of subject-matter knowledge. If you are not prepared to show *how* an interaction looks, there is not much point in testing for it, except of course to tell reviewers that you did test for proportional hazards.

Telling them that you did not bother to make a subject-matter-based inspection of the actual nature of the interactions is probably not a good idea.

Finally, testing for proportional hazards, i.e. interactions with the time-scale, naturally begs the question whether interactions between all the other variables in the models should be investigated. So cox.zph opens a can of worms for you.

8.6.3 *The Cox model as a Poisson model*

The Cox model can actually be seen as the limit of a rather special Poisson model. Suppose we subdivide the follow-up for all persons at all times of event or censoring, so that there is no change in risk set inside any interval, and that there is at most one death in each interval. The rates can then be analysed by using a Poisson model for these observations.

If instead of using a smooth parametric function for the baseline hazard we adapt a model with one parameter for each of these intervals, we will arrive at a model that is mathematically equivalent to the Cox model in the sense that it yields precisely the same estimates for the regression parameters as the Cox model. We will also have a lot of nuisance parameters (namely one per interval) that essentially just adds to the computing time.

```
> lung$time <- lung$time + runif( nrow(lung), -1, 1 )
> table( table(lung$time) )

  1
228
```

> CODE EXPLAINED: The event times (time) must all be distinct, so we add a small random quantity to the times to ensure this—runif generates random variables from the uniform distribution. The table(lung$time) will produce a table of the number of persons with each distinct time, so a table of 1s if no two identical times exist. Using table() on that table shows that the inner table actually only has entries of 1.

```
> L1 <- Lexis( exit = list(tfd = time),
+          exit.status = factor(status, labels = c("Alive","Dead")),
+              data = lung )
NOTE: entry.status has been set to "Alive" for all.
NOTE: entry is assumed to be 0 on the tfd timescale.
> cX <- coxph( Surv( tfd, lex.Xst=="Dead" ) ~ sex + age, data=L1 )
> cX <- coxph.Lexis( L1, tfd ~ sex + age )
survival::coxph analysis of Lexis object L1:
Rates for the transition Alive->Dead
Baseline timescale: tfd
```

> CODE EXPLAINED: The Lexis object is set up as previously, and the model fitted as before too, but now the data set has no two times identical.
>
> Once the Lexis object is defined, the wrapper coxph.Lexis can be used to simplify the fitting of a Cox model; the time-scale tfd must the be specified as the l.h.s. of the formula. The definition of events and risk time is automatically taken from the Lexis object.

```
> X1 <- splitMulti( L1, tfd=c(0,sort(unique(L1$time))) )
> summary( X1 )
```

```
Transitions:
     To
From    Alive Dead  Records:  Events: Risk time:  Persons:
  Alive 25941  165     26106      165   69590.09       228
> system.time(
+ pX <- glm( cbind(lex.Xst=="Dead",lex.dur) ~ factor(tfd) + sex + age,
+            family=poisreg, data=Xl ) )
   user  system elapsed
 53.685  57.416  31.064
> length( coef(pX) )
[1] 230
> rbind( ci.exp(cX),
+        ci.exp(pX,subset=c("sex","age")) )[c(1,3,2,4),]
      exp(Est.)       2.5%      97.5%
sexW  0.5997188  0.4319199  0.8327066
sexW  0.5997188  0.4319199  0.8327066
age   1.0172305  0.9990054  1.0357881
age   1.0172305  0.9990054  1.0357881
```

> CODE EXPLAINED: We use splitMulti from the popEpi package to subdivide the follow-up at all recorded times. Note we need to append 0 to the split points, because splitMulti ditches all follow-up outside the range of the split points given. We then fit a Poisson model to the split data, where we use a separate parameter for each of the 228 intervals (factor(tfd)). system.time measures the time that glm uses to fit the model. coef(pX) returns the estimates—there are 230 of them, one for each of the intervals plus the two regression parameters. Finally, ci.exp is used to extract the regression parameters from the two models, and rbind to stack them for comparison.

Thus we see that the Cox model regression estimates can be reproduced exactly by a quite silly Poisson model—namely, one with a separate parameter for each time recorded, 228 parameters on top of the two regression parameters. There is an awful lot of parameters in the Poisson model, and that is the reason it takes so long to fit—as seen from the system.time().

In section 8.6.1 we saw that using a penalized spline function to describe the baseline hazard would yield regression parameters very similar to those from the Cox model. So the conclusion is that the potential bias from using a Cox model is very small; as long as the interest is in the regression parameters only, the results from the two approaches are the same.

If the interest is in the survival curve, the approach with a smooth parametric model as outlined above gives more credible results, as seen from Figure 8.7.

8.7 Time-dependent covariates

If in the diabetes dataset we want to assess how much initiation of oral anti-diabetic drug (OAD) therapy (which starts at dooad) influences mortality rates, we must subdivide the follow-up by medication status. This means that we must subdivide the *follow-up* for the persons. Note that it is *not* a question of classifying *persons*; it is a classification of follow-up (time end events) into time before OAD and time after OAD. From a practical point of view this requires that some of the records in our dataset be split in two, and that we keep track of entry and exit times for each record.

For a person that initiates OAD at some point in time (dooad, that is), the time *before* is spent in the 'no OAD' and the time *after* in the 'OAD treated' state. In the practical analysis of data this requires that persons who change status be represented by two records.

The details of this have already been discussed in section 5.7, pp. 111, where Lexis objects for representation of follow-up data were introduced.

Briefly (very similar to what we did in 5.7), we define the follow-up structure in a Lexis object (note that we are including the duration of diabetes (tfd) as a time-scale too):

```
> Ldm <- Lexis( entry = list( tfd=0,
+                             age=dodm-dobth,
+                             per=dodm ),
+               exit = list( age=dox-dobth ),
+        exit.status = factor( !is.na(dodth), labels=c("Alive","Dead") ),
+               data = DMlate )
NOTE: entry.status has been set to "Alive" for all.
> Cdm <- cutLexis( data = Ldm,
+                   cut = Ldm$dooad,
+             timescale = "per",
+             new.state = "OAD",
+       precursor.states = "Alive" )
> oo <- options( digits=5 )
> subset( Ldm, lex.id %in% c(2,38) )[,c(1:7,10,12)]
        tfd    age    per lex.dur lex.Cst lex.Xst lex.id   dodm  dooad
307563    0 64.090 2003.3  6.6886   Alive   Alive      2 2003.3 2007.4
110338    0 63.932 2008.4  1.6318   Alive    Dead     38 2008.4 2008.7
> subset( Cdm, lex.id %in% c(2,38) )[,c(1:7,10,12)]
           tfd    age    per lex.dur lex.Cst lex.Xst lex.id   dodm  dooad
2      0.00000 64.090 2003.3 4.13689   Alive     OAD      2 2003.3 2007.4
9998   4.13689 68.227 2007.4 2.55168     OAD     OAD      2 2003.3 2007.4
38     0.00000 63.932 2008.4 0.30664   Alive     OAD     38 2008.4 2008.7
10034  0.30664 64.238 2008.7 1.32512     OAD    Dead     38 2008.4 2008.7
> options( oo )
> summary( Cdm )
Transitions:
     To
From   Alive  OAD Dead  Records:  Events: Risk time:  Persons:
  Alive 3292 3129 1208      7629     4337   26803.32      7629
  OAD      0 4205 1291      5496     1291   27469.95      5496
  Sum   3292 7334 2499     13125     5628   54273.27      9996
```

CODE EXPLAINED: The Lexis function creates a Lexis data frame with death as event and three time-scales: diabetes duration, tfd; current age, age; and calendar time, per. cutLexis cuts the follow-up (lex.dur,lex.Xst) at the time of oral anti-diabetic medication (dooad). The second record for each person has per equal to the date of OAD, and the outcome lex.Xst equal to the value in the original data Ldm. Also the sum of the risk time in lex.dur from the two records equals the total follow-up time in the original records. The argument precursor.states lists those states (in this case Alive), which will be over-written by the new state. So person 2 exits alive, so after starting OAD he remains in state OAD; however, person 38 exits dead, so after starting OAD he still exits dead, because Dead is *not* a precursor state.

The options(digits=5) restricts printing to 5 *significant* digits, and by assigning this to an object (oo), we can reset the options later by options(oo).

Each record in the Cdm dataset now represents an interval of follow-up. The variable tfd is the duration of diabetes at the start of the interval; age is the age at the start of the interval; per is the calendar time at the start of the interval; and lex.dur is the *length* of the interval.

A Cox model based on the expanded ('cut') dataset must be specified with the time-scale at the start (for example, tfd) and at the end of each interval (which then would be tfd + lex.dur). If we want to assess the effect of OAD on mortality we must refer to the lex.Cst variable—the indicator of where the person is during each interval of follow-up.

```
> ma <- coxph( Surv(tfd, tfd+lex.dur, lex.Xst=="Dead") ~ sex + lex.Cst,
+              data=Cdm )
```

CODE EXPLAINED: The Surv function takes an optional first of three arguments, namely the entry time, which in this case is the time-scale we use, tfd. The second argument is the exit time on this time-scale, which in this case is the time of entry *plus* the time spent before exit (sojourn time), lex.dur.

Since all the timing of the follow-up has been set up in the Lexis object, we have the possibility of simplifying the code via the wrapper coxph.Lexis:

```
> md <- coxph.Lexis( Cdm, formula = tfd ~ sex + lex.Cst )
survival::coxph analysis of Lexis object Cdm:
Rates for transitions Alive->Dead, OAD->Dead
Baseline timescale: tfd
> round( ci.exp(md), 2 )
            exp(Est.) 2.5% 97.5%
sexF             0.90 0.83  0.97
lex.CstOAD       1.06 0.98  1.15
lex.CstDead      1.00 1.00  1.00
```

CODE EXPLAINED: coxph.Lexis fits a Cox model to follow-up data in a Lexis object. The formula argument must have a time-scale on the l.h.s. of the ~ and the model formula on the r.h.s. It returns a coxph object.

The variable lex.Cst (Current state) is a factor with 3 levels (the same as lex.Xst, eXit state), namely Alive, OAD, and Dead, but the value Dead is never assumed by lex.Cst, but coxph does not automatically detect this, so a parameter estimate of NA is given, which by ci.exp is translated to a 1.

In principle we could show two survival curves from this model, one for persons not on OAD ('Alive') and on for persons on OAD ('OAD'):

```
> plot( survfit(md, newdata=data.frame(sex="M",lex.Cst="Alive")), yaxs="i" )
> lines( survfit(md, newdata=data.frame(sex="M",lex.Cst="OAD"  )), col="red" )
```

At first glance we see that the two curves (shown with confidence intervals) have the same pattern, and according to the results from the Cox model, persons on OAD have a higher

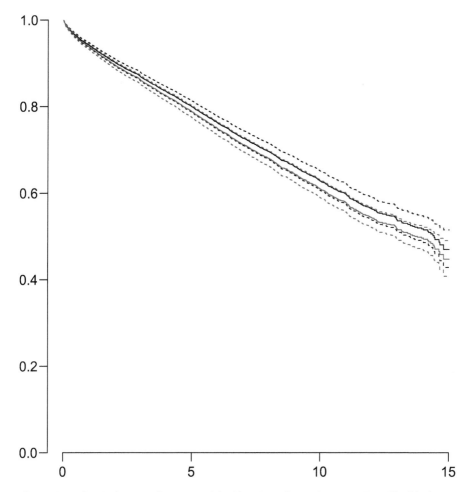

Figure 8.10 Survival curves from a model with a time-dependent covariate. The black curve is the survival among persons that will never go on OAD. The red curve is survival for persons who enter OAD *at* diagnosis. Neither make much sense.

mortality and hence a poorer survival. However, the black curve (Alive) is pure nonsense, while the red curve (OAD) is only partial nonsense.

The problem here is that we in the prediction treat the time-dependent covariate lex.Cst as if it were constant within each person, as if it represented a classification of *persons*. The black curve is showing the survival under the assumptions (1) that persons cannot transfer to OAD and (2) the mortality rate would be unchanged under that assumption [1, 2]. This is the so-called net-survival, or cause-specific survival; it has no probability interpretation in this world.

The red curve is the survival of persons who start on OAD immediately at diagnosis of diabetes, an event that actually does occur (approximately at least), even if the most common is that OAD initiation is some time after diagnosis. So it *is* a proper survival function, but it refers to a situation on the edge of the data.

So when we introduce a time-dependent covariate, such as OAD use, we lose the possibility of making a simple survival curve. But of course we can still ask questions, such as what is:

- the probability of being
  - alive at a given time
  - alive and not on OAD at a given time
  - alive and on OAD at a given time?
- the expected remaining time
  - alive
  - alive without OAD
  - alive with OAD?

...and how these depend on covariates.

These quantities do not only depend on the mortality rates of persons not on OAD and currently on OAD, but also on the rate with which persons switch to OAD. The latter has not been modelled here, so they cannot be quantified based on the models fitted here.

Estimation of these quantities is in the realm of multistate modelling, so is outside the scope of this book.

8.8 Competing risks

The following is not an exhaustive treatise on the concepts of competing risks, but only a brief introduction to the core concepts. You should not expect to be able to master the relevant techniques after reading this section. That would require the better part of a book about multistate models, and by that token is outside the scope of this book.

It is intended to warn you about the most common pitfalls. We shall again use the DMlate data on survival of Danish diabetes patients, where we also have information on the initiation of pharmaceutical treatment—dooad is the date of initiation of Oral Antidiabetic Drug.

If we want to assess how long newly diagnosed diabetes patients remain without pharmaceutical treatment, we must take into account those who die too. More precisely speaking we want to know what is the probability of being in each of the states: (1) remain alive without treatment (Alive) (2) being dead without any treatment (3) having initiated treatment, the latter regardless of subsequent death or not.

It is commonly seen that a survival curve is constructed from a model where transition to OAD is taken as event and deaths just counted as censorings. This is wrong; it will overestimate the probability of going on drugs. The standard reference for an overview of this is [1].

In the previous chapter we subdivided the follow-up into follow-up without OAD and follow-up after OAD. Here, we are only interested in persons who are initially without OAD treatment, so we restrict the Lexis data set Cdm to persons who are without OAD, that is, to persons in state Alive.

```
> Adm <- subset( Cdm, lex.Cst=="Alive" )
> summary( Adm )
Transitions:
     To
From    Alive  OAD Dead  Records:  Events: Risk time:  Persons:
  Alive  3292 3129 1208      7629     4337   26803.32      7629
> boxes( Adm, boxpos=list(x=c(50,20,80),y=c(80,20,20)),
+        scale.R=100, show.BE=TRUE )
```

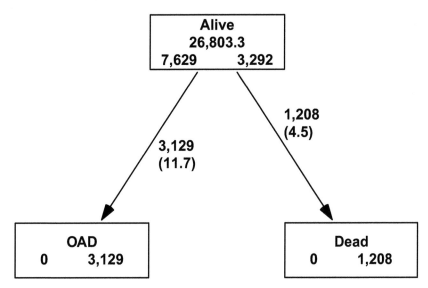

Figure 8.11 Transitions to Dead and OAD for Danish diabetes patients. The number in the middle of the box is the person-years; the numbers at the bottom of the boxes are the number of persons that begin, resp. end, their follow-up in each state. The numbers on the arrows are the number of transitions and the rates per 100 PY.

CODE EXPLAINED: First, we subset to the follow-up in the Alive state, and show how many transitions we have to Dead, resp. OAD. The function boxes.Lexis gives a graphical version of the summary; the boxpos argument determines the position of the boxes—the numbers refer to percentage of the plot extent; see Figure 8.11.

8.8.1 *Simple approach*

The survfit function has a facility that correctly estimates the probabilities of being in each state. It looks like a normal survival analysis but if the last argument to the Surv function is a factor, a proper estimation of the probabilities of being in each state will result. It is assumed that the first level corresponds to censoring, and the remaining levels to the possible types of events.

The question addressed by this competing risk analysis is the probability of starting drug treatment, and the OAD state here means 'having been on pharmaceutical treatment, disregarding subsequent death'. The other event considered is Dead which here means 'dead without initiating pharmaceutical treatment'.

```
> levels(Adm$lex.Xst)
[1] "Alive" "OAD"   "Dead"
> m3 <- survfit( Surv(tfd, tfd+lex.dur, lex.Xst) ~ 1,
+                data = Adm, id = lex.id )
> head( cbind( time = m3$time, m3$pstate ) )
            time
[1,] 0.002737851 0.9960676 0.002883733 0.001048630
[2,] 0.005475702 0.9909549 0.007472094 0.001573014
[3,] 0.008213552 0.9889885 0.008914151 0.002097398
[4,] 0.010951403 0.9876775 0.009700727 0.002621783
[5,] 0.013689254 0.9830891 0.014026896 0.002883975
[6,] 0.016427105 0.9796806 0.017042104 0.003277263
```

CODE EXPLAINED: Since lex.Xst is a factor, survfit will compute the Aalen–Johansen estimator of being in a given state and place the probabilities in the matrix m3$pstate; the times these refer to are in the vector m3$time.

You should try to explore the object m3 using names(m3)

The m3$pstate contains the Aalen–Johansen probabilities of being in the Alive state (green), having left to the OAD state (red), resp. Dead state (black). These three curves have sum 1, so basically this is a way of distributing the probabilities across states at each time.

It is therefore natural to stack the probabilities, which can be done by stackedCIF:

```
> par( mfrow=c(1,2) )
> matplot( m3$time, m3$pstate,
+          type="s", lty=1, lwd=4,
+          col=c("ForestGreen","red","black"),
+          ylim=c(0,1), yaxs="i" )
> stackedCIF( m3, lwd=3, yaxs="i" )
> text( rep(12,3), c(0.9,0.3,0.6), levels(Cdm) )
> box()
```

CODE EXPLAINED: par(mfrow=c(1,2)) defines a 1-by-2 layout of figures. The matplot plots the probabilities of being in each of the three states, Alive with green, OAD with red, and Dead with black.

In Figure 8.12, stackedCIF plots the stacked probabilities—the lower curve in the right plot is the same as the red in the left, the upper curve is the sum of the red and the black—the probability of being in either OAD or Dead, hence also 1 minus the probability of being in Alive (the green curve).

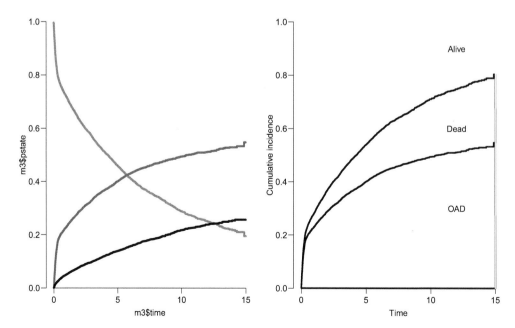

Figure 8.12 Separate state probabilities (left) and stacked state probabilities (right). (left) Alive is green, OAD is red and Dead is black.

8.8.2 *What not to do*

A very common error is to use a *partial* outcome such as OAD, when as in this case there is a competing type of event, Dead. If that is ignored and a traditional survival analysis is made *as if* OAD was the only possible event, we will have a substantial *over*estimate of the cumulative probability of going on the drug. Here is an illustration of this erroneous approach:

```
> m2 <- survfit( Surv(tfd,tfd+lex.dur,lex.Xst=="OAD") ~ 1, data=Adm )
> M2 <- survfit( Surv(tfd,tfd+lex.dur,lex.Xst=="Dead") ~ 1, data=Adm )
> par( mfrow=c(1,2) )
> mat2pol( m3$pstate, c(2,3,1), x=m3$time,
+          col=c("red","black","transparent"),
+          yaxs="i", xlab="time since DM", ylab="" )
>    lines( m2$time, 1-m2$surv, lwd=3, col="red" )
> mat2pol( m3$pstate, c(3,2,1), x=m3$time, yaxs="i",
+          col=c("black","red","transparent"),
+          yaxs="i", xlab="time since DM", ylab="" )
>    lines( M2$time, 1-M2$surv, lwd=3, col="black" )
```

> CODE EXPLAINED: The first two lines calculate the survival as if only OAD, respectively Dead, were the only way of exiting the state Alive. The mat2pol (matrix to polygon) takes the columns of state probabilities from the survfit object m3 that contains the correctly modelled probabilities and plots them as stacked areas. The second argument to mat2pol is the order in which they should be stacked. The lines plot the wrongly computed cumulative risks (from m2 and M2)—in order to find these we fish out the surv component from the survfit objects.

From Figure 8.13 we see that by ignoring the possibility of dying we will be substantially overestimating the probability of going on pharmaceutical treatment. The red curve is based on what is often termed the 'net' probability—it refers to the probability of OAD in a setting where (1) death does not occur and (2) the rate of pharmaceutical treatment is still the same in the absence of death.

A question frequently asked in competing risk situations is what is the probability of being on OAD, and it is often (wrongly) believed to be answered by the red curve in the left panel of Figure 8.13. But the highly unrealistic assumption (2) is often forgotten. How the rate of pharmaceutical treatment would look in the absence of death (or vice versa for that matter) cannot be deduced from data where both types of risk are present. It is essentially a theological question as no data are available.

8.8.3 *A mathematical explanation*

Suppose the rate of drug initiation (Alive→OAD) is $\lambda(t)$ and the mortality before drug initiation (Alive→Dead) is $\mu(t)$; then the probability of being alive without drug treatment at time t is

$$S(t) = \exp\left(-\int_0^t \lambda(s) + \mu(s)\,\mathrm{d}s\right) \tag{8.2}$$

and the cumulative risk of initiating drug before time t is

$$R_{\mathrm{OAD}}(t) = \int_0^t \lambda(u)S(u)\,\mathrm{d}u = \int_0^t \lambda(u)\exp\left(-\int_0^u \lambda(s) + \mu(s)\,\mathrm{d}s\right)\mathrm{d}u \tag{8.3}$$

—and similarly for the cumulative risk of death (just swap λ and μ).

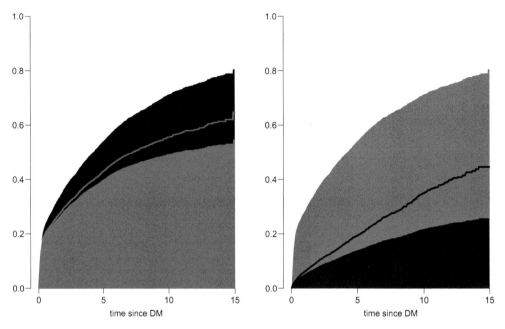

Figure 8.13 Stacked state probabilities. `Alive` is white, `OAD` is red, and `Dead` is black. The red line in the left panel is the wrong (but often computed) 'cumulative risk' of `OAD`, and the black line in the right panel is the wrong (but often computed) 'cumulative risk' of `Death`. The black and the red areas in the two plots represent the correctly computed probabilities; they have the same size in both panels; only they are stacked differently.

The error committed in the analysis pretending that only the event `OAD` is present is *not* in the calculations of the cause-specific rates; it is *only* in the calculations of the cumulative risk (probability of transition to `OAD`). The red line in Figure 8.13 comes from omitting the term $\mu(s)$ from formula (8.3). The temptation is apparently that if you do that, the mathematics becomes nicer:

$$R_{\text{OAD}}(t) = \int_0^t \lambda(u)\exp\left(-\int_0^u \lambda(s)\,\mathrm{d}s\right)\mathrm{d}u = 1 - \exp\left(-\int_0^t \lambda(s)\,\mathrm{d}s\right) \qquad (8.4)$$

and this is precisely what comes out of standard programs when regarding `OAD` as the only type of event.

So there is no such thing as a competing risk analysis of event *rates*; the competing risks aspect comes about only when you want to address the cumulative risk of a particular event. In which case you probably want to look at the cumulative risks of all types of events.

8.9 Modelling cause specific rates

As we just saw, there is nothing wrong with modelling the cause-specific event rates; the problem lies in how you transform them into probabilities.

As above we can model the two sets of rates by a parametric model; this must be based on a time-split data set:

```
> Sdm <- splitMulti( Adm, tfd=seq(0,20,0.1) )
> summary(Sdm)
Transitions:
     To
From     Alive  OAD Dead   Records:   Events: Risk time:  Persons:
  Alive 267536 3129 1208     271873      4337   26803.32       7629
> gl <- gam.Lexis( Sdm, ~ s(tfd), from="Alive", to="OAD" )
mgcv::gam Poisson analysis of Lexis object Sdm with log link:
Rates for the transition: Alive->OAD
> gm <- gam.Lexis( Sdm, ~ s(tfd), from="Alive", to="Dead" )
mgcv::gam Poisson analysis of Lexis object Sdm with log link:
Rates for the transition: Alive->Dead
```

We can derive the estimated rates from the two models for rates by time by using prediction frames:

```
> int <- 0.01
> nd <- data.frame( tfd=seq(int,15,int)-int/2 )
> mrt <- ci.pred( gm, nd )[,1]
> lam <- ci.pred( gl, nd )[,1]
```

The vectors mrt and lam now contain the two rates evaluated at the midpoint of intervals of length int=0.01 years. Since the variable lex.dur is in units of years, the rates are in units of events per 1 person-year.

We then translate formulae (8.2) and (8.3) directly into computer code, using the fact that an integral is just a sum, and since we want the integrals as functions of the upper limits we use cumsum, remembering to multiply by the interval length:

```
> Lam <- cumsum( lam * int )       # cumulative incidence of OAD
> Mrt <- cumsum( mrt * int )       # cumulative mortality
> Srv <- exp( -( Mrt+Lam ) )       # survival in Alive state
> crO <- cumsum( lam * Srv * int ) # cumulative risk of OAD
> crD <- cumsum( mrt * Srv * int ) # cumulative risk of Death
```

Now we have the survival (in Alive) in Srv and the cumulative risks in crO and crD.

```
> matplot( m3$time, m3$pstate,
+          type="s", lty=1, lwd=1,
+          col=c("ForestGreen","red","black"),
+          ylim=c(0,1), yaxs="i" )
> matlines( nd$tfd, cbind( Srv, crO, crD ),
+          type="l", lty="21", lwd=3, lend="butt",
+          col=c("ForestGreen","red","black") )
```

From Figure 8.14 we see that the results from the two approaches are pretty much the same: the smoothed curve gives a bit higher value for the probability of being on the drug around 1 year.

There is nothing wrong with the estimate of the *rate* of initiating drugs. It is only the calculation of the survival *probability* that is wrong—the probability of having initiated a drug depends on *both* the rate of drug initiation *and* the mortality rate, that is, on all of the rates *out* of the Alive box in Figure 8.11.

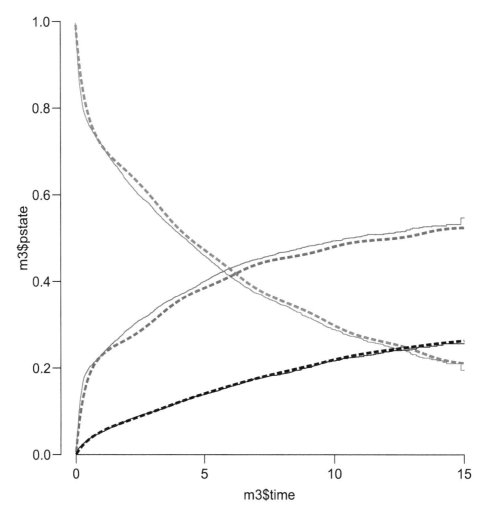

Figure 8.14 Comparison of the non-parametric estimates of the state probabilities (thin lines) with the probabilities based on gam-smoothed rates (broken lines).

8.9.1 *Limitations*

The parametric approach produces more credible estimates than does the non-parametric approach, but as seen here, the approach relies on the availability of explicit formulae. In practice this means that competing risk models can be treated, but that more complicated multistate models cannot be reported using this approach.

Neither of the approaches here will deal with models where rates depend on multiple time-scales, particularly on time-scales defined as time since entry to an intermediate state (such as mortality depending on the time since drug initiation or on the time between diagnosis and drug initiation). This type of results can essentially only be derived using simulation; you may want to consult the vignette on this in the Epi package:

```
> vignette("simLexis","Epi")
```

8.10 The Fine–Gray approach to competing risks

Fine and Gray [5] defined models for the subdistribution hazard, $\tilde{\lambda}_i(a)$. To this end, recall the relationship between between the hazard (λ) and the cumulative risk (F):

$$\lambda(a) = -\frac{\mathrm{d}\log(S(a))}{\mathrm{d}a} = -\frac{\mathrm{d}\log(1 - F(a))}{\mathrm{d}a}$$

When more competing causes of death are present the Fine–Gray idea is to use this transformation to the cause-specific cumulative risk for cause 1, say:

$$\tilde{\lambda}_1(a) = -\frac{\mathrm{d}\log(1 - F_1(a))}{\mathrm{d}a}$$

The quantity $\tilde{\lambda}_1$ is called the subdistribution hazard; as a function of $F_1(a)$ it depends on the survival function S, which depends on *all* the cause-specific hazards:

$$F_1(a) = P\{\text{dead from cause 1 at } a\} = \int_0^a \lambda_1(u)S(u)\,\mathrm{d}u$$

The subdistribution hazard is merely a transformation of the cause-specific cumulative risk. Namely the same transformation which in the single-cause case transforms the cumulative risk to the hazard. It is a purely mathematical construct, and it is not interpretable as a hazard despite its name.

The Fine–Gray approach is a non-parametric model for a mathematical transform of *one* cause-specific cumulative risk, controlling for all other types of competing events.

If we model each of the competing hazards by the Fine–Gray approach, it turns out that there is no guarantee that the sum of the predicted cumulative risks will be 1—the Fine–Gray model is not a model for the entire set of competing hazards; it is designed to give an estimate of the cumulative risk of one type of event controlling for other competing events. You can find an illustration of this odd behaviour in the vignette on competing risks in the `survival` package:

```
> vignette( "compete", "survival" )
```

As opposed to this, if we base calculations on models for each cause-specific hazard separately we will get results that have the property that the sum of the estimated probabilities of being in any of the states is 1, just as most people prefer to think reality behaves.

8.11 Time-dependent variables and competing risks

The analysis of Dead using the OAD as a time-dependent variable and the analysis of Dead and OAD as competing risks address different aspects of a *multistate model*, the illness-death model, which is is illustrated in Figure 8.15 (in two different guises).

Here is how we arrive at these plots:

```
> par( mfrow=c(1,2), cex=0.5 )
> boxes( Cdm, boxpos = list(x=c(20,80,50),
+                           y=c(80,80,20)),
+         scale.R=100, show.BE=TRUE )
> Xdm <- cutLexis( data = Ldm,
+                   cut = Ldm$dooad,
+              timescale = "per",
```

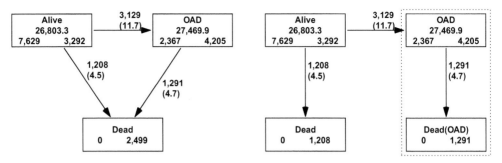

Figure 8.15 The illness–death model with initiations of OAD as illness state. In the left panel we do not distinguish according to the state before death, as is done in the right panel. The box within the dotted line is the state OAD used in the competing risk analysis. The number in the middle of each box is the person-years; the numbers at the bottom of the boxes are the number of persons that begin, resp. end, their follow-up in each state. The number a on the arrows are the number of transitions and the rates per 100 PY.

```
+               new.state = "OAD",
+        precursor.states = "Alive",
+            split.states = TRUE )
> boxes( Xdm, boxpos = list(x=c(20,80,20,80),
+                           y=c(80,80,20,20)),
+        scale.R=100, show.BE=TRUE )
> rect( 61,8,99,92, lty=3, lwd=2 )
```

CODE EXPLAINED: boxes plot state-boxes for the dataset Cdm, the argument boxpos giving the position of the boxes (in % of the plot extent). This gives an illustration of an illness–death model, with three states and three transitions.

If we want to distinguish dead persons by whether they were on OAD at death, we must subdivide the Dead state by the state prior to Dead. This is done by adding split.states=TRUE to the cutLexis function, which will produce a Lexis object (Xdm) where the Dead state is subdivided by the state from which death occurs, so with 4 states. The boxpos argument to boxes will therefore need vectors of length 4.

When we are using OAD as a time-dependent variable we are modelling the two mortality rates Alive→Dead and OAD→Dead, ignoring the rates of OAD (Alive→OAD). The simplest model just assumes that the two mortality rates are proportional.

In the analysis of competing risks, only the rates Alive→Dead and Alive→OAD are modelled, and then used to derive the probability of being in each of three states, Alive, Dead *without* OAD, and OAD *or* dead after OAD. The latter is illustrated by the dotted box in the right panel of Figure 8.15.

If we use models for all three rates we would be able to derive probabilities of being in any of the four states illustrated in the right panel of Figure 8.15. This can be done mathematically and translated to code but it is not a pretty sight. If you want to do that sort of thing you will most likely have to resort to simulation methods and an extensive introduction to multistate modelling, which is outside the scope of this book.

The Epi package does contain some tools for this, described in two vignettes; try:

```
> vignette( "flup", "Epi" )
> vignette( "simLexis", "Epi" )
```

CHAPTER 9

Do not group quantitative variables

The following section is a direct quote from the website of Vanderbilt University's Department of Biostatistics, http://biostat.mc.vanderbilt.edu/CatContinuous, explaining the problems flowing from categorization.

The department kindly allowed me to include it here. In the text you will find further links to articles describing the problems with categorizing quantitative variable (here termed *continuous* variables).

9.1 Problems Caused by Categorizing Continuous Variables

1. Optimum decisions are made by applying a utility function to a predicted value (e.g. predicted risk). At the decision point, one can solve for the personalized cutpoint for predicted risk that optimizes the decision. Dichotomization on independent variables is completely at odds with making optimal decisions. To make an optimal decision, the cutpoint for a predictor would necessarily be a function of the continuous values of all the other predictors, as shown in Section 18.3.1 of http://hbiostat.org/doc/bbr.pdf.
2. Loss of power and loss of precision of estimated means, odds, hazards, etc. Dichotomization of a predictor requires the researcher to add a new predictor to the mix to make up for the lost information.
3. Categorization assumes that the relationship between the predictor and the response is flat within intervals; this assumption is far less reasonable than a linearity assumption in most cases
4. Researchers seldom agree on the choice of cutpoint; thus there is a severe interpretation problem. One study may provide an odds ratio for comparing BMI>30 with BMI≤ 30, another for comparing BMI>28 with BMI≤ 28. Neither of these has a good definition and they have different meanings.
5. Categorization of continuous variables using percentiles is particularly hazardous. The percentiles are usually estimated from the data at hand, are estimated with sampling error, and do not relate to percentiles of the same variable in a population. Percentiling a variable is declaring to readers that how similar a person is to other persons is as important as how the physical characteristics of the measurement predict outcomes. For example, it is common to group the continuous variable BMI into quantile intervals. BMI has a smooth relationship with every outcome studied, and relates to outcome according to anatomy and physiology and not according to how many subjects have a similar BMI.

Epidemiology with R. Bendix Carstensen, Oxford University Press (2021). © Bendix Carstensen.
DOI: 10.1093/oso/9780198841326.003.0010

6. To make a continuous predictor be more accurately modelled when categorization is used, multiple intervals are required. The needed dummy variables will spend more degrees of freedom than will fitting a smooth relationship; hence power and precision will suffer. And because of sample size limitations in the very low and very high range of the variable, the outer intervals (e.g. outer quintiles) will be wide, resulting in significant heterogeneity of subjects within those intervals, and residual confounding.

7. Categorization assumes that there is a discontinuity in response as interval boundaries are crossed.

8. Categorization only seems to yield interpretable estimates such as odds ratios. For example, suppose one computes the odds ratio for stroke for persons with a systolic blood pressure >160 mmHg compared to persons with a blood pressure ≤160 mmHg. The interpretation of the resulting odds ratio will depend on the exact distribution of blood pressures in the sample (the proportion of subjects >170, >180, etc.). On the other hand, if blood pressure is modelled as a continuous variable (e.g. using a regression spline, quadratic, or linear effect) one can estimate the ratio of odds for *exact* settings of the predictor, e.g. the odds ratio for 200 mmHg compared to 120 mmHg.

9. When the risk of stroke is being assessed for a new subject with a known blood pressure (say 162), the subject does not report to her physician 'my blood pressure exceeds 160' but rather reports 162 mmHg. The risk for this subject will be much lower than that of a subject with a blood pressure of 200 mmHg.

10. If cutpoints are determined in a way that is not blinded to the response variable, calculation of P-values and confidence intervals requires special simulation techniques; ordinary inferential methods are completely invalid. For example, if cutpoints are chosen by trial and error in a way that utilizes the response, even informally, ordinary P-values will be too small and confidence intervals will not have the claimed coverage probabilities. The correct Monte-Carlo simulations must take into account both multiplicities and uncertainty in the choice of cutpoints. For example, if a cutpoint is chosen that minimizes the P-value and the resulting P-value is 0.05, the true type I error can easily be above 0.5; see https://onlinelibrary.wiley.com/doi/abs/10.1002/sim.1611

11. Likewise, categorization that is not blinded to the response variable results in biased effect estimates (see https://academic.oup.com/jnci/article-abstract/86/11/829/955201?redirectedFrom=fulltext and http://repository.essex.ac.uk/2513/)

12. 'Optimal' cutpoints do not replicate over studies. Hollander, Sauerbrei, and Schumacher (see https://onlinelibrary.wiley.com/doi/abs/10.1002/sim.1611) state that 'the optimal cutpoint approach has disadvantages. One of these is that in almost every study where this method is applied, another cutpoint will emerge. This makes comparisons across studies extremely difficult or even impossible. Altman et al. point out this problem for studies of the prognostic relevance of the S-phase fraction in breast cancer published in the literature. They identified 19 different cutpoints used in the literature; some of them were solely used because they emerged as the 'optimal' cutpoint in a specific data set. In a meta-analysis on the relationship between cathepsin-D content and disease-free survival in node-negative breast cancer patients, 12 studies were included with 12 different cutpoints ...Interestingly, neither cathepsin-D nor the S-phase fraction are recommended to be used as prognostic markers in breast cancer in the recent update of the American Society of Clinical Oncology.'

13. Cutpoints are arbitrary and manipulatable; cutpoints that can result in both positive and negative associations can be found (see https://www.tandfonline.com/doi/abs/10.1080/09332480.2006.10722771)

14. If a confounder is adjusted for by categorization, there will be residual confounding that can be explained away by inclusion of the continuous form of the predictor in the model in addition to the categories.

15. A better approach that maximizes power and that only assumes a smooth relationship is to use a restricted cubic spline (regression spline; piecewise cubic polynomial) function for predictors that are not known to predict linearly. Use of flexible parametric approaches such as this allows standard inference techniques (P-values, confidence limits) to be used.

References

[1] P. K. Andersen, R. B. Geskus, T. de Witte, and H. Putter. Competing risks in epidemiology: possibilities and pitfalls. *International Journal of Epidemiology*, Jan 2012.

[2] P. K. Andersen and N. Keiding. Interpretability and importance of functionals in competing risks and multistate models. *Statistics in Medicine*, 31:1074–1088, 2012.

[3] B. Carstensen. Age–period–cohort models for the Lexis diagram. *Statistics in Medicine*, 26(15): 3018–3045, July 2007.

[4] B. Carstensen and M. Plummer. Using Lexis objects for multi-state models in R. *Journal of Statistical Software*, 38(6):1–18, 2011.

[5] J. P. Fine and R. J. Gray. A proportional hazards model for the subdistribution of a competing risk. *Journal of the American Statitical Association*, 94:496–509, 1999.

[6] A. Bradford Hill. The environment and disease: association or causation? *Proceedings of the Royal Society of Medicine*, 1965.

[7] J. A. Nelder and R. W. M Wedderburn. Generalized linear models. *Journal of the Royal Statistical Society (A)*, 135(10):370–384, 1972.

[8] C. Osmond and M. J. Gardner. Age, period, and cohort models. Non-overlapping cohorts don't resolve the identification problem. *American Journal of Epidemiology*, 129(1):31–35, 1989.

[9] M. Plummer and B. Carstensen. Lexis: an R class for epidemiological studies with long-term follow-up. *Journal of Statistical Software*, 38(5):1–12, 2011.

Index